The Essentials of Pediatrics

The Essentials of Pediatrics
The Clinical Core in Outline

ARTHUR J. MOSS, M.D.

Professor of Pediatrics,
University of California at Los Angeles
School of Medicine,
Los Angeles, California

THOMAS J. MOSS, M.D.

House Officer in Pediatrics,
Children's Hospital of Los Angeles,
Los Angeles, California

J. B. Lippincott Company
PHILADELPHIA
London—Mexico City—New York
St. Louis—São Paulo—Sydney

5 6 4

Library of Congress Cataloging in Publication Data

Moss, Arthur J
   The essentials of pediatrics.

   Bibliography:
   Includes index.
   1. Pediatrics—Outlines, syllabi, etc. I. Moss,
Thomas J., joint author. II. Title. [DNLM:
1. Pediatrics—Outlines. WS18 M913e]
RJ48.3.M67   618.92   80-15301
ISBN 0-397-50466-7

The authors and publisher have exerted every
effort to ensure that drug selection and dosage set
forth in this text are in accord with current recommendations and practice at the time of publication. However, in view of ongoing research,
changes in government regulations, and the constant flow of information relating to drug therapy
and drug reactions, the reader is urged to check
the package insert for each drug for any change
in indications and dosage and for added warn-
ings and precautions. This is particularly important when the recommended agent is a new or
infrequently employed drug.

Contents

Preface

Pediatrics is that branch of medicine which relates to the growth and development of infants and children and to their care in health and disease. Age groups currently embraced include the *neonate*, the *infant*, the *preschool child*, the *school-age child*, and the *adolescent*.

Standard textbooks on this subject have become so detailed and so voluminous that they cannot possibly be absorbed in their entirety. As a result, they are used principally as ready references for a particular subject, and they are usually an excellent source for that purpose. There is a need, however, for more compact and less detailed texts for those who wish to survey in the shortest possible time only the fundamentals of general pediatrics.

This book is designed to fulfill such a purpose. It is intended, in large measure, to satisfy the needs of the medical student who may or may not pursue a career in pediatrics. Family practitioners, pediatricians, pediatric house officers, nurses, and others who deal with children may also find it useful for quick review. The material represents a broad overview or "core" knowledge of pediatrics and is not meant to be a comprehensive or detailed dissertation on the subject. For example, dosages and specifics of treatment, for the most part, are deleted, since this information is usually readily available from other sources. Also, in the interest of brevity and simplicity, a number of the less common and more esoteric disorders are not included.

The outline type of format is used because it permits the widest coverage of a broad subject in the smallest space and should appeal to those who wish to cover quickly the basic aspects of health and disease in infants, children, and adolescents.

Arthur J. Moss, M.D.
Thomas J. Moss, M.D.

The
Essentials of
Pediatrics

1

History and Physical Examination

HISTORY

A. Source
   1. Parent, sibling, other relative, neighbor, or friend
   2. Estimate reliability of source
B. Present Complaint (PC)
   Age, race, sex, and brief statement regarding present complaint
C. Present Illness (PI)
   Detailed and specific discussion of initial and subsequent symptoms with dates, pertinent negative data, history of exposure for acute infections
D. Past History
   1. Antenatal
      Pertinent data relating to previous health of mother, to illnesses or abnormal symptoms during pregnancy, roentgenographic procedures, medications
   2. Natal
      a. Birth weight
      b. Gestational period
      c. Duration of labor, type of delivery, sedation and anesthesia, resuscitation

3. Neonatal

   Cyanosis, convulsions, jaundice, fever, ability to suck, congenital abnormalities, birth injury, duration of hospital stay

4. Development
   a. When head up, rolled over, sat alone, crawled, stood alone, first words, urinary continence at night and during day, control of feces, first tooth
   b. Comparison of development with siblings
   c. Age started school, scholastic and social achievement

5. Nutrition
   a. Breast or formula (type, duration)
   b. Type and duration of vitamin supplements
   c. When solid foods introduced
   d. Appetite; food likes, dislikes, idiosyncracies

6. Immunization and tests
   a. Type, number, age
   b. Specific interrogation regarding tetanus, diphtheria, pertussis, measles, rubella, mumps, poliomyelitis, tuberculin testing, boosters

7. Habits and personality

   Aggressive, hyperactive, enuresis, encopresis, sleep problems, tics, pica,* nail-biting, thumb-sucking

8. Illnesses, operations, injuries
   a. Infections
   b. Contagious diseases—measles, mumps, pertussis, rubella, chickenpox
   c. Date and place of operation
   d. Accidents and injuries—type, time, extent

9. Family history

   Siblings, consanguinity, cause of deaths and at what age, allergies, blood dyscrasias, tuberculosis, heart disease, obesity, convulsions, nervous diseases, diabetes, congenital abnormalities

10. Social history
    a. Size of home and family, neighborhood, play facilities
    b. Occupation of parents
    c. Who provides care for patient
    d. Third-party coverage

11. Review of systems
    a. Eyes, ears, nose, throat
       1. Tearing, strabismus; redness, itching of eyes
       2. Colds, sore throats, sneezing, snoring, mouth breathing, nasal discharge, otitis, hearing
    b. Cardiopulmonary
       Wheezing, cough, cyanosis, edema, syncope, palpitations
    c. Gastrointestinal

* See Glossary

       Abdominal pain, diarrhea, vomiting, constipation, melena,*
       hematemesis,* jaundice
  d. Genitourinary
       Pyuria, hematuria, urethral discharge, vaginal discharge, menstrual ab-
       normalities, dysuria, polyuria, bladder control
  e. Neuromuscular
       Paralysis, paresis, tremors, gait, exercise tolerance, postural deformities
  f. Endocrine
       Polyphagia,* polydipsia,* pattern of growth, thyroid disease, menarche,
       unusual weight gain or loss

PHYSICAL EXAMINATION

A. General Considerations
  1. Record temperature, pulse, respirations
  2. Record blood pressure
  3. Record height, weight (absolute numbers and percentiles)
  4. Calculate surface area
  5. Record head circumference (absolute numbers and percentile) in infants and,
     when indicated, in older children
B. General Appearance
    State of nutrition, cry, distress, gait, position, attitude, level of consciousness,
    facies, facial expression
C. Approach to the Examination
  1. *Slow* and friendly
  2. May have to undress child piecemeal
  3. Wash hands in warm water
  4. Leave ear, nose, and throat examination for last
  5. Warm stethoscope with hands
D. Skin
  1. Cyanosis, jaundice, pallor, flushing, warmth
  2. Turgor, edema, elasticity
  3. Nevi, pigmentation, eruptions, striae, hemangiomas
E. Lymph Nodes
    Size, mobility, consistency
F. Head
    Size, shape, circumference, fontanelles, sutures, venous distention, bruits,
    transillumination
G. Neck
    Position, masses, thyroid size, thyroid nodules, thyroid bruit, webbing, move-
    ment, tonic neck reflex

* See Glossary

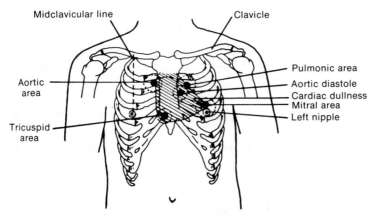

Fig. 1. Listening areas of the heart. (*Reproduced with permission from Barness LA: Manual of Pediatric Physical Diagnosis, 4th edition. Copyright © 1972 by Year Book Medical Publishers, Inc., Chicago*)

H. Thorax

Asymmetry, dilated veins, rib flaring, sternal deformity, intercostal retractions, substernal retractions, epigastric retractions, Harrison's grooves,* size and location of nipples

I. Lungs

1. Limitation of motion on either side
2. Dullness or flatness to percussion
3. Rales, rhonchi, wheezes, fremitus

J. Heart (Fig. 1)

1. Location and intensity of apex beat, thrills, ventricular heave and thrust
2. Rate, rhythm, systolic clicks,* intensity of heart sounds, friction rub, murmurs (location, intensity, systolic or diastolic, transmission)
3. Percussion of no value in infants and small children because 1-cm error can mean the difference between normal size heart and cardiomegaly

K. Abdomen

1. Peristaltic waves, venous distention, hernias, musculature
2. Tenderness, rigidity, shifting dullness, rebound tenderness, liver, spleen, other organs or masses
3. Bowel sounds
4. Infants may have to be examined in mother's lap or while taking a bottle

L. Eyes, Ears, Nose, Throat

1. *Eyes:* Ptosis,* epicanthal folds, Mongolian slant, lacrimation, photophobia, nystagmus, strabismus, opsiclonus,* size and reactivity of pupils, conjunctiva, sclera, enophthalmus,* corneal clouding or opacities, cataracts, Brushfield spots,* aniridia,* heterochromia,* fundoscopic, vision

* See Glossary

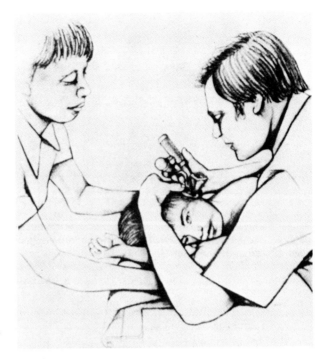

Fig. 2. Otoscopic examination of the child. (*Hoekelman RA: In Bates B: A Guide to Physical Examination, p. 341. Philadelphia, Lippincott, 1974*)

2. *Ears:* Deformity, position, discharge, foreign body, tympanic membrane, hearing (Fig. 2)
3. *Nose:* Patency of nares, obstruction, discharge, septal deviation or perforation, turbinates, polyps
4. *Mouth and throat:* Lips, tongue, number of teeth, dental caries, dental discoloration, buccal and gingival mucosa, enanthem,* stenotic orifices, uvula, tonsils, pharynx (Fig. 3)
5. With infants and young children, restraint may be necessary

M. Genitalia
1. *Male:* Hypospadias, epispadias, chordee,* phimosis, cryptorchidism, size of testes, scrotum, hernia, hydrocele,* circumcision, meatus, pubertal changes (see Chap. VIII)
2. *Female:* External examination only unless otherwise indicated and rarely before puberty. Vulva, clitoris, discharge, pubertal changes

N. Rectum and Anus
1. Fissures, prolapse, imperforate
2. Digital examination carried out with use of little finger in infants and small children
3. Muscle tone, masses, tenderness, presence of stool, character of stool

* See Glossary

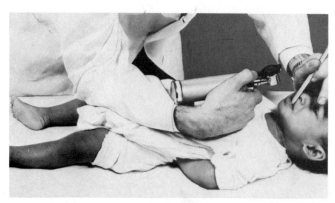

Fig. 3. Restraining the patient for examination of the mouth. Patient's arms are tucked under his back. Examiner's hand presses on chest and holds light. Examiner's other hand holds patient's head and tongue depressor (*Reproduced with permission from Barness, LA: Manual of Pediatric Physical Diagnosis, 4th edition. Copyright © 1972 by Year Book Medical Publishers, Inc., Chicago*)

O. Extremities
    1. Deformity, asymmetry, edema, paresis, paralysis, limitation of motion, swelling, redness, pain, carrying angles,* temperature, simean creases
    2. Cyanosis, clubbing, pulsations
P. Back
    Posture, spinal curvature, mongolian spots,* tenderness, pilonidal dimple or sinus or cyst, sensation

BIBLIOGRAPHY

Barness LA: Manual of Pediatric Physical Diagnosis. Chicago, Year Book, 1966

Hoekelman RA et al: Principles of Pediatrics. Health Care of the Young. New York, McGraw-Hill, 1978

Kempe CH, Silver HK, O'Brien D: Current Pediatric Diagnosis and Treatment. Los Altos, Lange, 1976

Rudolph AM, Barnett HL, Einhorn AH: Pediatrics. New York, Appleton-Century-Crofts, 1977

Vaughan VC III, McKay RJ, Nelson WE: Nelson Textbook of Pediatrics. Philadelphia, W. B. Saunders, 1975

* See Glossary

2 | The Newborn Infant

CARE IN DELIVERY ROOM

A. Gentle Suction of Oral Cavity with Soft Rubber Bulb Syringe to Remove Mucus
B. Apgar Score at 1 and 5 Minutes (Table 1) to Document Appraisal of Physical Condition
C. Warm Environment to Prevent Heat Loss
D. Examine Baby and Placenta
E. 1% Silver Nitrate in Eyes for Prophylaxis Against Gonorrhea
F. Transfer to Nursery (Preferably in Heated Incubator)

CLASSIFICATION

A. Full Term:
    Is 38–42 weeks gestation and usually more than 2500 g birth weight and less than 3750 g
B. Small for Gestational Age (SGA):
    Synonyms are small-for-date, intrauterine growth retardation. Birth weight less than 10th percentile

TABLE 1 Apgar Score* for Evaluation of Newborn

PHYSICAL CONDITION	SCORE
Heart rate	
Absent	0
Less than 100	1
Over 100	2
Respiratory effort	
Absent	0
Slow, irregular	1
Lusty cry	2
Muscle tone	
Limp	0
Some extremity flexion	1
Active	2
Response to catheter in nostril	
None	0
Grimace	1
Cough or sneeze	2
Color	
Blue	0
Pale	0
Blue, extremities only	1
Pink	2

* Total score of 10 indicates that baby is in best possible condition.

C. Premature:

Less than 38 weeks gestation. Usually less than 2500 g birth weight

D. Postmature:

Gestation greater than 42 weeks

PHYSICAL CHARACTERISTICS

A. Weight and Body Measurements of Full Term Infant
 1. Birth weight 2500–3750 g
 2. Length 48–50 cm
 3. Initial postnatal weight loss regained by 10 days of age
 4. Head circumference at birth is 32–37 cm. Serial measurements are important
 5. Average weight gain 4–6 ounces per week in early months
B. Activity

Responds to stimulation by movement and lusty cry

C. Skin
 1. Vernix caseosa* covering at birth

* See Glossary

2. Fine downy hair on forehead and face (lanugo). More pronounced in premature infants
3. Visible sebaceous glands on nose (milia) (Fig. 4)
4. Transient acrocyanosis* normally present
5. Occasional petechiae not abnormal
6. In dark-skinned races, bluish areas on back and sometimes on extremities not uncommon (Mongolian spots) (Fig. 5)
7. Mottling of skin common in premature and small-for-gestational-age babies
8. Telangiectasis* over eyelids, glabella,* mid forehead, lumbosacral area, and nape of neck common. Usually disappear by 2 years of age
9. Maculopapular transient dermatitis (erythema toxicum) requires no treatment. Disappears within first week (Fig. 6)
10. Premature infant has thin shiny skin with little or no subcutaneous fat. Also, extremities may be edematous
11. Postmature infants often have loss of subcutaneous tissue, desquamation of skin and meconium staining (Fig. 7)

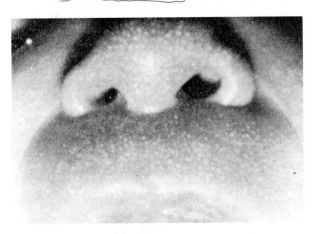

Fig. 4. Hyperplastic sebaceous glands in the nasolabial region and a solitary epidermal inclusion cyst (milium) on the right cheek of a term infant. Note the disparity in size between the milium and the sebaceous glands. (*Hodgman JE et al: Neonatal dermatology. Pediatr Clin North Am 18:713, 1971*)

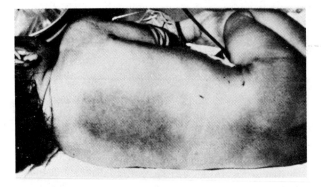

Fig. 5. Mongolian spots. (*Phibbs RH: In Rudolph AM, Barnett HL, Einhorn AH (eds): Pediatrics, p. 145. New York, Appleton-Century-Crofts, 1977*)

* See Glossary

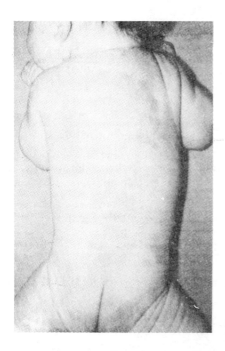

Fig. 6. Common distribution of typical lesions of toxic erythema in a 24-hour-old term infant. (*Hodgman JE et al: Neonatal dermatology. Pediatr Clin North Am 18:713, 1971*)

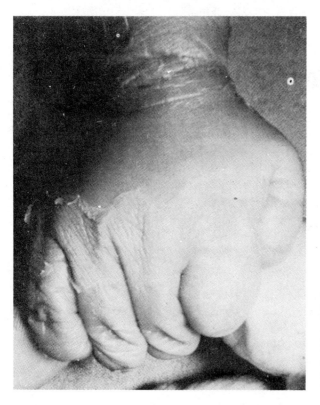

Fig. 7. Hand of a dysmature term infant at 4 hours of age. The collodianlike epidermis has peeled from the fingers, revealing skin markings. (*Hodgman, JE et al: Neonatal dermatology. Pediatr Clin North Am 18: 713, 1971*)

       12. Creases on sole of foot and rugae on scrotum are less pronounced or absent in premature infants

D. Head (Fig. 8)
    1. Anterior and posterior fontanelles are open
    2. Sagittal, coronal, lambdoidal sutures are open
    3. Occiput may be transiently misshapen as a result of edema (caput succedaneum) consequent to labor and delivery (molding) (Fig. 9)
    4. Thin area of calvarium that may be slightly indented with pressure (like a Ping-Pong ball) may be normally present (craniotabes)

E. Eyes
    1. Transient edema of eyelids from instillation of silver nitrate common
    2. Episcleral and conjunctival hemorrhages not uncommon
    3. Iris not fully pigmented for as long as one year
    4. White specks in iris seen in 20–30% of normal babies
    5. Fundoscopic examination requires use of mydriatic (1 drop of 10% Neosynephrine HCl in each eye). Often not successful

F. Ears
    Some cartilage present

G. Mouth and Pharynx
    1. Mucus-retention cysts normally present on palate (Epstein's pearls)
    2. Teeth rarely present
    3. High arched palate may be normal

H. Chest
    1. Respiratory rate may normally be up to 50–60/min
    2. Supernumerary nipples of no significance
    3. Breast tissue present in normal term infants

I. Heart and Lungs
    1. Percussion of no value
    2. Normal heart rate 100–160/min
    3. Soft systolic murmurs common. Require observation since some persist and are significant. Most disappear spontaneously
    4. Second sound in pulmonic area—normally loud and single during early hours of life

J. Abdomen
    1. Liver may normally be palpated 2 cm below costal margin
    2. Spleen tip may be normally felt
    3. Kidneys may be normally palpated

K. Genitalia
    1. Prepuce cannot be fully retracted but can be pushed back to reveal meatus
    2. Testes may not be palpable in premature infant
    3. Hydrocele of little or no clinical significance in newborn
    4. Labia minora and clitoris prominent in premature infant
    5. Vaginal bleeding during first week not uncommon (estrogen withdrawal phenomenon)

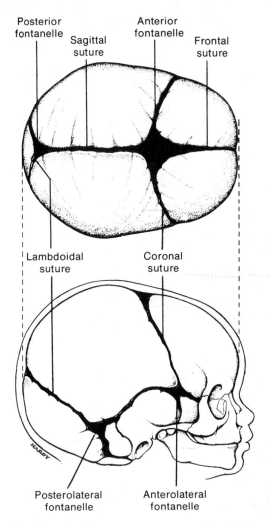

Posterior
fontanelle

Sagittal
suture

Anterior
fontanelle

Frontal
suture

Lambdoidal
suture

Coronal
suture

HARDY

Posterolateral
fontanelle

Anterolateral
fontanelle

Fig. 8. Normal fontanelles in newborn infant that may be palpated or visualized roentgenographically. (*Chaffee EE, Lytle IM: Basic Physiology and Anatomy, 4th ed., Philadelphia, J. B. Lippincott, 1980*)

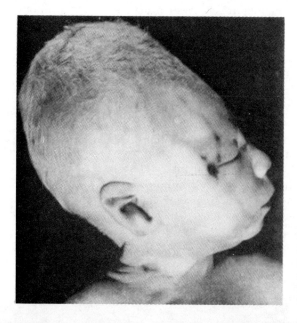

Fig. 9. Head molding with caput succedaneum over vortex. (*Reproduced with permission from Potter EL, Craig JM: Pathology of the Fetus and the Infant, 3rd edition. Copyright © 1975 by Year Book Medical Publishers Inc., Chicago*)

L. Extremities

    Mild syndactyly* of second and third toes normal

M. Reflexes

1. *Recoil:* After stretching and release of extremity, it returns to flexed position
2. *Suck:* Normally present at birth
3. *Ankle clonus:* Common and not significant if unsustained
4. *Knee jerk:* Moderately brisk
5. *Babinski:* Often positive in normal infants
6. *Moro* (abduction of upper arms, extension of elbows and opening of fists with sudden noise, jarring, lifting body and head, or hyperextension of neck): Normally present to 4 months of age
7. *Rooting:* Head turns in direction of stimulation of mouth or cheeks
8. *Grasp:* Closes fist when palm is stimulated
9. *Righting:* When infant is lifted off examining surface and soles of feet are allowed to touch table, legs extend, then trunk and head
10. *Automatic walking:* When infant is lifted off examining surface and soles of feet are kept in contact with table, a "walking" motion of legs occurs

FEEDING IN NEONATAL PERIOD

A. Breast Feeding

1. Is the ideal nutrient
2. To be successful, mother must *want* to breast feed
3. Five minutes on each breast beginning first day. By 3–4 days, this should be increased to 10 minutes on each breast
4. Feed every 2½–3 hours during first week, then every 2½–4 hours. Do not wake baby during night to feed
5. Water necessary only on very warm days

B. Artificial Feeding

1. Same schedule as above
2. Offer 2–4 ounces per feeding—to be increased by about 1 ounce per month up to 8 ounces
3. Total duration of sucking should not exceed 20 minutes
4. Baby should be held while feeding—*bottle should not be propped* or air swallowing could occur
5. Water necessary only on very warm days
6. Premature and small-for-gestational-age infants should be given smaller amounts at more frequent intervals (*i.e.,* q 2 h). Gavage* or parenteral feedings may be necessary for very small infants
7. A variety of formulas available (Enfamil, Similac, SMA)
8. Formula selected should be isocaloric with breast milk (20 cal/oz)

* See Glossary

VITAMIN AND MINERAL SUPPLEMENTS

A. If Formula Contains Vitamins, Added Vitamins Not Necessary
B. If Vitamin Intake is Less Than 500 IU for A, 400 IU for D, and 20 mg for C, Vitamin Supplements Should be Started at 2 Weeks
C. Vitamins C and D Beginning at 2 Weeks to Breast-Fed Babies
D. Iron Supplementation Started No Later Than 2 Months in Premature Infants and 4 Months in Term Infants. Cow's Milk is Poor Source. May be Provided by Iron-fortified Milk or by Daily Administration of Ferrous Sulfate Drops (1 mg/kg/day for term infants and 2 mg/kg/day for premature infants—maximum dose 15 mg/day)
E. Fluoride Supplement (0.5 mg daily) if Drinking-Water Content is Less Than 1 Part Per Million

CARE OF PREMATURE INFANT

A. May Require Incubator to Maintain Body Temperature
B. Body Temperature Should Be Maintained at About 36°C
C. Start Feedings at 2–4 Hours if Condition Permits
D. Start With Oral Glucose Solution and Gradually Increase Amounts and Replace With Formula
E. Have Increased Need for Vitamins C and D (50 mg vitamin C and 1000 IU vitamin D daily beginning at 2–3 weeks)
F. Hand-Scrubbing Technique Must be Rigidly Observed
G. Use of Increased Ambient Oxygen To Be Avoided (for fear of retrolental fibro-plasia*) Unless Condition Requires It

CLINICAL DISORDERS OF NEWBORN

A. Birth Defects
  Congenital malformations (general considerations)
  a. Account for 15% of neonatal deaths
  b. Incidence of major malformations is 3–4%, of minor malformations, 14%
  c. Due to gene mutation (*i.e.*, Hurler's disease), chromosomal abnormalities (*i.e.*, Down's syndrome), unfavorable intrauterine environment (*i.e.*, rubella syndrome)
  d. Known patterns of associated malformations sometimes occur, such as VATER syndrome, (vertebral anomalies, anal atresia, tracheoesophageal fistula, renal anomalies)
  e. High-risk mothers include older mothers (more than 35 years), those with unfavorable genetic background, infection or exposure to teratogenic drugs and toxic agents, diabetes, polyhydramnios,* oligohydramnios*

* See Glossary

f. *Minor* malformations not handicapping and require no treatment. These include epicanthal folds, upward slant of palpebral fissures (mongoloid slant), Brushfield spots, low-set ears, rotated ears, preauricular tags or pits, simian line (single horizontal palmar crease), clinodactyly (lateral deformity of fingers), camptodactyly (flexion deformity of fingers), single umbilical artery

(handwritten: white spots on iris ~ Down's syn)

1. If three or more, than a major malformation is present in 90%
2. Require careful search for major malformations

g. *Major* malformations require careful search for associated abnormalities, referral to appropriate center, and genetic counseling. Specific malformations discussed in subsequent sections related to specific organs or tissue

h. Indications for chromosome studies
1. Three or more malformations (major or minor)
2. Mental retardation plus two or more malformations
3. Moderate mental retardation
4. Known chromosome disorder such as Down's syndrome
5. Ambiguous external genitalia
6. Short stature in females
7. Failure to develop secondary sex changes
8. Male hypogonadism

B. Some of the More Common Specific Infections
1. Intrauterine infections (TORCH group)
   a. IgM may be elevated in all (indicates *intrauterine* infection only if elevated during first day or two)
   b. Toxoplasmosis
      1. *Features:* Microcephaly, small for date, hydrocephaly, cerebral calcifications, chorioretinitis
      2. *Other manifestations:* Encephalitis, diarrhea, vomiting, jaundice, convulsions, myocarditis, hepatomegaly, splenomegaly
      3. *Laboratory diagnosis:* Specific antibody titers
      4. *Treatment:* Sulfadiazine
   c. Rubella syndrome
      1. *Features:* Microcephaly, small for date, glaucoma, cataracts, retinopathy, microphthalmia, congenital heart disease
      2. *Other manifestations:* Hepatomegaly, splenomegaly, hepatitis, thrombocytopenia, petechial rash (Fig. 10) pneumonia, myocarditis, encephalitis, osteitis *(handwritten: Blueberry muffin rash)*
      3. *Laboratory diagnosis:* Antibody titers, viral cultures from throat, urine, spinal fluid
      4. *Treatment:* Symptomatic only. Must be isolated
   d. Cytomegalovirus
      1. *Features:* Microcephaly, small for date, cerebral calcifications
      2. *Other manifestations:* Like those for toxoplasmosis
      3. *Laboratory diagnosis:* Antibody titers, viral cultures from throat, urine, spinal fluid

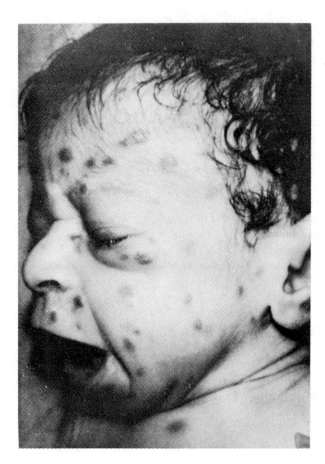

Fig. 10. Blueberry muffin lesions in an undergrown term infant with congenital rubella who died at 1 week of age. (*Hodgman JE et al: Neonatal dermatology. Pediatr Clin North Am 18:713, 1971*)

    e. Herpes simplex
        1. Features: Chorioretinitis, microcephaly, microphthalmia, small for date
        2. Other manifestations: Skin vesicles, hepatitis, encephalitis
        3. Laboratory diagnosis: Antibody titers, cultures from vesicles, throat, urine, spinal fluid
        4. Treatment: Adenine arabinoside (Ara-A)
  2. Congenital infections other than TORCH group
    a. Syphilis
        1. Features: Late involvement of eyes, ears, teeth, joints, central nervous system, Hutchinson triad*
        2. Other manifestations: Osteochondritis, periostitis, rhagades,* anemia, hepatomegaly, splenomegaly, cutaneous lesions, nephritis, nephrosis, rhinitis, ("snuffles")

* See Glossary

        3. *Laboratory diagnosis:* Dark-field examination, nontreponemal tests (VDRL), fluorescent treponemal antibody absorption (FTA-ABS)

        4. *Treatment:* Aqueous procaine penicillin G

   b. Gonococcal infection

        1. *Features:* Conjunctivitis, panophthalmitis, sepsis

        2. *Laboratory diagnosis:* Gram stain and culture

        3. *Treatment:* Aqueous penicillin G

   c. Coxsackie B infection

        1. *Features:* Encephalomyocarditis, pneumonia

        2. *Laboratory diagnosis:* Antibody titers, cultures from throat, feces, cerebrospinal fluid

        3. *Treatment:* Symptomatic only

3. Postnatal infections in neonate

   a. Neonatal sepsis and meningitis

        1. *Agents:* Escherichia coli, Klebsiella, Enterobacteriaceae, serratiae, protei, pseudomonads, listeriae, flavobacteria, streptococci, (mainly group B), Mima polymorphia, Hemophilus influenzae, penumococcus, meningococcus, staphylococcus. E. coli and group B streptococci account for 70%

        2. *Onset:* Usually during first 3 days. Group B streptococcal meningitis may be delayed for 1–2 weeks

        3. *Manifestations:* Poor cry, poor suck, lethargy, poor feedings, hypothermia, hyperthermia, convulsions, jaundice, hepatomegaly, splenomegaly

        4. *Laboratory diagnosis:* Cultures from all possible infected sites including blood, urine, cerebrospinal fluid

        5. *Treatment*

           a. Appropriate antibiotic according to agent and sensitivities

           b. Treat for 10–14 days (14–21 days if meningitis is associated)

           c. Oxygen, parenteral fluids, nasogastric suction as necessary

           d. Blood transfusions if anemic

           e. Repeat blood cultures 24–48 hours after initiation of treatment and 48 hours after antibiotics are discontinued

           f. Measure head size daily during therapy and on follow-up visits to detect subdural effusion, subdural empyema, hydrocephalus

           g. Isolate for first 24–48 hours

   b. Chlamydial infections

        1. Agent is *Chlamydia trachomatis*

        2. Infection acquired from maternal genital tract during delivery

        3. Presents as conjunctivitis and/or pneumonia. May become apparent weeks or months after birth

        4. May produce chronic pertussislike cough

        5. Fever usually absent

        6. Eosinophilia often present

        7. *Laboratory diagnosis:* Fluorescent antibody titers, cultures from conjunctivae, nasopharynx, tracheal aspirate

       8. *Treatment:* For *conjuctivitis,* local instillation of 10% sulfacetamide ointment or 1% tetracycline ointment. For *pneumonia,* sulfisoxazole or erythromycin

  c. Group B streptococcal infection

      1. *General considerations:* Primary reservoir is maternal genitourinary tract. Four types of organisms

      2. *Manifestations:* Early overwhelming pneumonia (all 4 types) or late meningitis (usually type IV) and sepsis 1 week to several months after birth

      3. *Treatment:* Supportive, penicillin

      4. *Prognosis:* Pneumonic type usually runs rapid course with 40–80% mortality. Meningitis type carries 15–20% mortality

  d. Impetigo

      1. Lesions in neonate are vesicular or bullous

      2. Due to Staphylococcus aureus*

      3. Treatment includes isolation, oxacillin

C. Birth Injuries

  1. Cephalhematoma (Fig. 11)

    a. Is *subperiosteal* hemorrhage, so *never* crosses suture line

    b. No skin discoloration

    c. Swelling may not be visible for several hours

    d. With time, rim becomes organized giving sensation of central depression suggesting a depressed fracture

    e. May begin to calcify at 2 weeks and remain for months

    f. Should *not* be aspirated

    g. Requires no specific treatment

    h. Differs from encephalocele† in that latter involves suture line and increases in size and tension with crying

  2. Intracranial hemorrhage

    a. Due to anoxia, trauma, rarely to hemorrhagic diathesis or cerebral vascular anomaly

    b. More common in breech deliveries, precipitate deliveries, mechanically assisted deliveries. Also more common in premature infants, distressed infants

    c. *Manifestations:* Symptoms may be present at birth or appear hours or days later. May have lethargy, somnolence, absent Moro reflex, irregular respirations, apnea, pallor, cyanosis, poor suck, vomiting, irritability, twitchings, convulsions, bulging fontanelle, unequal pupils, retinal hemorrhages, failure of pupils to react, nystagmus

    d. *Diagnosis:* Subdural tap, lumbar puncture, transillumination, cerebral computer tomography (CT scan)

---

  * In older infants and children, lesions are frequently due to streptococcus infection and are crusted or purulent. Penicillin V or intramuscular benzathine penicillin G is antibiotic of choice

  † See Glossary

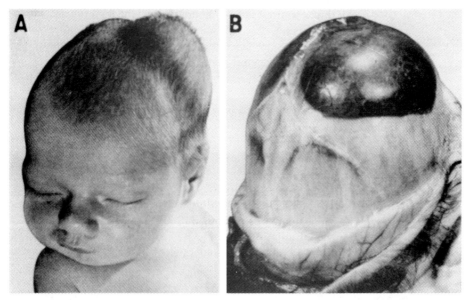

Fig. 11. Cephalhematoma over left parietal bone. **(A)** External view in living infant. **(B)** Scalp reflected to show localization of blood to subpericranial area. (*Reproduced with permission from Potter EL, Craig JM: Pathology of the Fetus and the Infant, 3rd edition. Copyright © 1975 by Year Book Medical Publishers, Inc., Chicago*)

     e. *Treatment:* Symptomatic. Repeated subdural taps for subdural hemorrhage. In selected cases of intraventricular, subarachnoid or intracerebral hemorrhage, repeated spinal fluid drainage for relief of increased intracranial pressure believed by some to be indicated

     f. *Prognosis:* Guarded, but may recover completely

  3. Spinal injuries

     a. More common in breech deliveries

     b. Usually at level of cervical vertebra 7 or thoracic vertebra 1

     c. Injury consists of hemorrhage, edema, or transection of cord

     d. With hemorrhage and edema, paralysis may be *transient;* with transection, paralysis is *permanent*

  4. Neuromuscular injuries

     a. Brachial palsy

        1. *Erb-Duchenne paralysis:* Injury involves fifth and sixth cervical nerves. Unable to abduct upper arm or supinate forearm

        2. *Klumpke's paralysis:* Injury involves seventh and eighth cervical and first thoracic nerves. Symptoms include hand paralysis and ipsilateral* ptosis and miosis* if first thoracic nerve is involved

        3. Prognosis and treatment

* See Glossary

        a. Good if injury is just edema or hemorrhage—function returns within a few months

        b. Guarded if nerves are lacerated—paralysis may be permanent

        c. Immobilization of affected part

        d. Consider neuroplasty if paralysis persists beyond 3–6 months

   b. Phrenic nerve paralysis

      1. Causes diaphragmatic paralysis with cyanosis and dyspnea

      2. Diagnosis established by fluoroscopy

      3. Recovery usually spontaneous but surgical plication of diaphragm may be necessary in occasional case

   c. Facial nerve palsy

      1. More common in forceps deliveries

      2. Improvement usually occurs within a few weeks. With laceration of nerve, neuroplasty may be necessary

   d. Sternocleidomastoid muscle injury

      Hemorrhage or laceration causes contracture of muscle with appearance of small firm nodule*

  5. Visceral Injuries

   a. Commonly due to overzealous resuscitation attempts

   b. Include rupture of liver or spleen

   c. Adrenal hemorrhage may be due to anoxia, trauma

   d. Surgical repair of liver or spleen lacerations may be necessary

  6. Fractures

   a. Clavicle most frequent. Prognosis excellent. Often first recognized by lump of callus on clavicle at 1- to 2-week examination

   b. Fractures of extremities require immobilization

D. Anoxia

  1. *Manifestations:* Meconium-stained amniotic fluid, pallor, cyanosis, apnea, bradycardia, flaccidity, failure to respond to mechanical stimulation

  2. *Treatment:* Clearing of airways, mechanical stimulation, and, if necessary, cardiopulmonary resuscitation. If Apgar score is less than 3 or if pulse rate is less than 80/min, artificial respiration or pulmonary inflation is usually indicated. Oxygen administered first by mask and, if ineffective, by endotracheal intubation (after lower respiratory passages are suctioned)

E. Electrolyte Disturbances and Other Neonatal Disorders

  1. Hypocalcemia

   a. May occur in prematurity, infants of diabetic mothers, birth asphyxia, sepsis, respiratory distress syndrome. Serum calcium less than 7.5 mg/100 ml but ionized portion must be less than 4 mg/100 ml. If seizures or apnea occurs, intravenous calcium gluconate indicated (2–3 ml/kg of a 10% solution)

   b. *Neonatal tetany†* occurs later (end first week or beginning of second). Presents with muscle twitching or seizures. Occurs almost exclusively in

---

* Requires early passive stretching to prevent torticollis (lateral tilting of head)
† See Glossary

artificially fed infants—high phosphate load depresses calcium level. Treatment includes administration of 10% calcium gluconate (2–3 mg/kg intravenously or orally). Parathyroid hormone reverses trend

    c. Chvostek* and Trousseau* signs may be positive in normal infants and are not reliable signs of hypocalcemia. Serum calcium *must* be measured to establish diagnosis

2. Hypoglycemia

    a. Occurs mainly in infants of diabetic mothers, intrauterine growth retardation, hypoxia, erythroblastosis fetalis

    b. *Signs:* Jitteriness, tremors, lethargy, high-pitched cry, poor suck, cyanosis, flaccidity or seizures

    c. *Diagnosis:* Based on two abnormal readings as follows: below 20 mg/dl for infants less than 2500 g; below 30 mg/dl for term infants less than 72 hours; below 40 mg/dl after 72 hours

    d. *Treatment of infant of diabetic mother:* Glucagon, epinephrine if asymptomatic. If symptomatic, glucose orally or intravenously. If no response to foregoing, hydrocortisone

    e. *Treatment in intrauterine growth retardation* includes early feedings, glucose, hydrocortisone as described previously

3. Idiopathic respiratory distress syndrome (RDS) (hyaline membrane disease)

    a. *General considerations:* Occurs mainly in premature infants and infants of diabetic mothers. Is most important life-threatening illness of newborn

    b. *Etiology:* Not established but evidence indicates lack of pulmonary surfactant

    c. *Manifestations:* Shortly after birth. Tachypnea, chest retractions, flaring of alae nasi, cyanosis, apnea, hypotension, peripheral edema, hypothermia, grunting, normal or slow heart rate, poor peripheral perfusion. Intracranial hemorrhage frequently associated. Intermittent systolic murmur may reflect opening and closing of ductus arteriosus. May be fatal with death usually in first 2–3 days. Course may be prolonged and terminate in bronchopulmonary dysplasia

    d. *Diagnosis:* Clinical manifestations, low Pa_{O_2}, acidemia, low lecithin : sphingomyelin ratio in tracheal aspirate, hyperkalemia, "ground-glass" appearance of lungs on roentgenogram

    e. *Treatment:* Maintenance of Pa_{O_2} at 60–80 mm Hg, mechanical ventilation if severe, neutral thermal environment, blood transfusion for hypotension, intravenous fluids, correction of acid–base imbalance and electrolyte disturbance

    f. *Prediction of RDS:* By determination of lecithin : sphingomyelin ratio of amniotic fluid (>2.0 means minimal risk)

    g. *Associated patent ductus arteriosus:* If signs of heart failure are present with no response to decongestive measures, surgical ligation or pharmacologic closure by administration of indomethacin may be indicated

* See Glossary

    h. *Bronchopulmonary dysplasia* is a complication that may be due to ventilator, to oxygen therapy, or to both. Precise cause not established. Roentgenogram shows honeycomb lesions with areas of lucency and density. Often reversible and many infants recover full pulmonary function after weeks, months, occasionally years

4. Meconium aspiration
    a. *General considerations:* Associated with high morbidity and mortality. Meconium-stained amniotic fluid earliest sign. Skin, umbilical cord, and nails may be meconium stained
    b. *Manifestations:* Mild to severe respiratory distress. Roentgenogram shows diffuse infiltration and hyperaeration. Pneumomediastinum, pneumothorax may be present
    c. *Treatment:* Supportive. Steroids not helpful

5. Persistent pulmonary hypertension
    a. *General considerations:* Also referred to as persistent fetal circulation, persistent pulmonary vascular obstruction, progressive pulmonary hypertension, persistent transitional circulation, persistence of fetal cardiopulmonary circulatory pathway
    b. *Manifestations:* Early cyanosis, tachypnea, acidemia, normal lung fields on roentgenogram, normal heart on roentgenogram. Systolic murmur may be audible. May have right-to-left shunting through patent ductus arteriosus demonstrable by heart catheterization
    c. *Treatment:* Supportive. Tolazoline may be helpful
    d. *Prognosis:* Guarded

6. Hyperbilirubinemia
    a. *Physiologic*
        1. Develops *after 24* hours of life
        2. Serum bilirubin not more than 12 mg/dl in term infants or 15 mg/dl in premature infants
        3. Cause unknown but probably related to increased hemolysis plus immaturity of liver
        4. Almost never produces symptoms
        5. Bilirubin reaches maximum at 2–4 days of age and becomes normal by 7–14 days of age in term infants—somewhat later in premature infants
        6. Bilirubin is indirect
        7. Other conditions must be excluded so should determine blood group and Rh of mother and baby, perform Coombs' test* on baby, total and direct bilirubin measurement, hemoglobin, hematocrit, peripheral blood smear, reticulocyte count, leukocyte count, urinalysis
    b. *Erythroblastosis fetalis (hemolytic disease of newborn)*
        1. *Mechanism:* Rh negative mother is sensitized by previous blood transfusion or by transplacental passage of Rh positive cells from Rh positive fetus during previous pregnancy. Transplacental passage of anti-Rh

* See Glossary

antibody to fetus of future pregnancies causes isoimmune hemolytic anemia in fetus

2. *Rh negative prevalence:* 15% of Caucasians, 5% of blacks, and virtually 0% of orientals are Rh negative. (Rh negative refers to D antigen. C and E antigens are also on same gene locus)

3. *Other considerations:* Analysis of bilirubin in amniotic fluid permits evaluation of severity of disease in fetus and is helpful in determining whether *intrauterine* transfusion is indicated. Sensitization of Rh negative mothers may be prevented by administration of anti-Rh antibody (RhoGAM) within 72 hours after each delivery of an Rh positive baby. Affected baby may be delivered of an Rh *positive* mother if sensitization is to the C or E antigens (rare) rather than to the D antigen. Disease may also be due to ABO incompatibility (passage of anti-A or anti-B antibodies from group O mother to group A or B fetus)

4. *Detection of sensitization: Indirect* Coombs' test is agglutination test on mother's serum for presence of antibodies. *Direct* Coombs' test is on baby's serum

5. *Manifestations*
   a. *Hepatomegaly* and *splenomegaly* are reflections of increased hematopoiesis
   b. *Hyperbilirubinemia* is reflection of liver damage
   c. *Hypoglycemia* is reflection of hyperinsulinism
   d. *Hydrops fetalis* (massive anasarca) is reflection of hypoalbuminemia, increased capillary fragility, or heart failure (Fig. 12)
   e. *Anemia* is reflection of hemolysis. Erythroblasts may be as high as 100,000/cu ml. Reticulocytes range from 15% to 80%. *Thrombocytopenia* common. Purpura and brain or pulmonary hemorrhage may occur
   f. *Respiratory distress* not uncommon

6. *Management*
   a. Supportive
   b. *Prevention of kernicterus:* Correct hypoalbuminemia by infusion of salt-poor albumin. Control hyperbilirubinemia by phototherapy in mild cases but in moderate or severe disease, exchange transfusion is a must. Indications for exchange transfusion not clearly defined, but rate of rise of unconjugated bilirubin greater than 1 mg/hour considered dangerous. Thus, bilirubin levels must be monitored closely (every 2–4 hours if rate of rise is rapid). Exchange transfusion consists of 2 volume exchange (twice the estimated blood volume of infant). Blood volume of infant is estimated on basis of 85 ml/kg body weight. Rh negative group O blood should be used
   c. *Hypoglycemia:* Dextrostix testing indicated at frequent intervals until carbohydrate intake is sufficient to ensure stable blood levels
   d. *Late care:* Anemia may develop during early months of life and may be severe enough to require transfusion

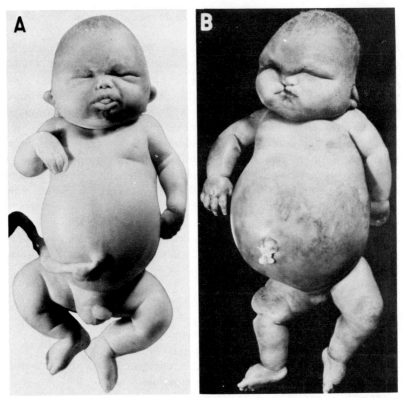

Fig. 12. Generalized anasarca. **(A)** Fetus stillborn because of erythroblastosis. **(B)** Fetus without erythroblastosis but with multiple malformations. (*Reproduced with permission from Potter EL, Craig JM: Pathology of the Fetus and the Infant, 3rd edition. Copyright © 1975 by Year Book Medical Publishers, Inc., Chicago*)

7. *ABO hemolytic disease:* Have little antibody so Coombs' test is only weakly positive. In contrast to Rh sensitization, disease tends to become milder with succeeding pregnancies rather than more severe. Disease generally mild with little or no anemia at birth and only mild hyperbilirubinemia. Phototherapy or exchange transfusions usually not required

c. *Breast-feeding jaundice:* Hyperbilirubinemia develops at 4–7 days in about 0.5% of breast-fed infants. Unconjugated bilirubin levels may reach 25 mg/dl. May persist for as long as 10 weeks but interruption of nursing for 6–9 days returns bilirubin level to normal. Resumption of nursing causes only small rise. Infants with this disease are asymptomatic and nursing need not be interrupted unless bilirubin level exceeds 20 mg/dl. Disorder is due to inhibition of glucuronyl transferase by pregnanediol in breast milk. Other causes must be excluded

d. *Jaundice due to hemorrhage:* Collection of large amounts of blood in body of infant can result in large loads of unconjugated bilirubin that liver cannot completely clear, conjugate, and excrete in bile

e. *Sepsis:* An important cause of hyperbilirubinemia

f. *Hepatitis:* Jaundice usually appears at 1–6 weeks of age but may be present at birth. Both conjugated and unconjugated fractions of bilirubin are increased. May be due to infectious agent such as hepatitis B virus, toxoplasma, syphilis, cytomegalovirus, Listeria, rubella virus, herpesvirus, varcella virus, coxsackie virus. Liver function tests are abnormal. Must be differentiated from biliary atresia, and this often requires exploratory operation and liver biopsy. Most infants recover with just supportive therapy

g. *Glucose-6-phosphate dehydrogenase (G6PD) deficiency*
   1. Sex-linked recessive (X chromosome)
   2. More common in blacks (10%). Also common in oriental and Mediterranean infants
   3. Manifest by episodes of acute hemolysis that are characterized by pallor, jaundice, and even shock and death. Episodes are precipitated by ingestion of certain drugs or other hemolytic agents
    4. G6PD deficiency results in failure to recycle reduced glutathione, which protects red-cell components from oxidation
   5. Diagnosis established by quantitative assay of enzyme activity in red-cell lysates

h. *Galactosemia*
   1. *General considerations:* Inborn error of galactose metabolism in which galactose-1-phosphate uridyl transferase is lacking or galactokinase is deficient
   2. *Manifestations:* Prior to milk feedings, baby is asymptomatic. Thereafter, hepatomegaly, jaundice, vomiting, diarrhea, lethargy, hypotonia, weight loss, and sometimes death. Cataracts may appear early
   3. *Diagnosis:* Galactose in urine, not detected by testape or clinitest; Fehling's or Benedict's test is necessary. Enzyme assay for transferase is definitive test
   4. *Treatment:* Immediate elimination of lactose or galactose from diet
   5. *Prognosis:* Manifestations disappear with treatment. Normal growth pattern may be achieved with proper dietary management. The earlier the treatment, the better the results

i. *Biliary atresia:* May be intra or extrahepatic. Jaundice appears at 1–6 weeks. Have complete biliary obstruction with acholic stools,* bilirubin in urine. Serum bilirubin level does not usually exceed 12 mg/dl in early months of life but rises later. Must be differentiated from neonatal hepatitis. This may be possible only by exploratory operation, liver biopsy, and cholangiography. If amenable to surgery, must be performed early before obstructive biliary cirrhosis appears (by 3–4 months). Most are inoperable, and death usually occurs before end of second year.

* See Glossary

j. *Complications of hyperbilirubinemia*

Kernicterus

a. *Definition:* Yellow staining of basal ganglia in infants with hyperbilirubinemia

b. *Etiology:* Unconjugated bilirubin destroys neural tissue. Unconjugated bilirubin is bound to albumin, and kernicterus occurs when albumin cannot bind enough unconjugated bilirubin

c. *Manifestations:* Initial symptoms between second and fourth days of life include lethargy, poor suck, slow Moro reflex, hypotonia. Hypotonia replaced by rigidity followed by extraocular muscular paresis (setting-sun sign),* twitching, oculogyric crises,* and convulsions. Death in 50% of full term and 75% of premature newborns. Survivors usually have choreoathetosis,* rigidity, high-frequency deafness, and/or faulty tooth enamel formation

d. *Prevention:* Phototherapy and exchange transfusion

7. Infant of diabetic mother

a. Macrosomia* and visceromegaly frequent. Babies large, puffy, and fat at birth—often over 4000 g

b. Extramedullary erythropoiesis common

c. Increased incidence of venous thrombosis, especially of renal veins

d. Hyaline membrane disease common

e. Major congenital malformations occur in 5% and may involve any organ system

f. Hypoglycemia commonly present (insulin levels elevated)

g. Hypercalcemia and hyperbilirubinemia may occur

h. Treatment is supportive with particular attention to hypoglycemia

i. May suffer from transient cardiomyopathy

j. Major problem and principal cause of death is respiratory distress syndrome

k. Mother may have no overt signs of diabetes mellitus but may be in prediabetic stage. When babies with foregoing manifestations are encountered, mother should have blood sugar and glucose tolerance test

8. Fetal alcohol syndrome

a. Offspring of alcoholic mothers may suffer from variety of congenital defects—no fixed pattern

b. Manifestations include short palpebral fissures, epicanthal folds, micrognathia,* low nasal bridge, long upper lip, narrow vermillion border, and flattened philtrum. Abnormal palmar creases, ear anomalies, cardiac defects may be present. Midfacial hypoplasia (maxillary flattening) may be observed. Baby often small for gestational age

c. Cardiac defects in about 40% of cases and are most often ventricular or atrial septal defects

d. Baby may show withdrawal symptoms (tremors, irritability, increased muscle tone, increased respiratory rate, arching of back, seizures)

* See Glossary

e. Postnatal growth deficiency, microcephaly, developmental delay, mental deficiency have also been observed
9. Retrolental fibroplasia (RLF)
   a. A retinopathy that may remain stationary or regress in early stages or may proceed to progressive cicatricial disease with eventual retinal detachment. In advanced cases, a dense white mass forms behind lens, producing total blindness
   b. Although reported in full term infants, prematurity is considered fundamental with excess oxygen the major precipitating or aggravating factor
   c. Safe level of arterial PO_2 not yet determined but levels should certainly not exceed 100 mm Hg
   d. May occur without oxygen administration. Both vitamin E deficiency and exchange transfusions have been incriminated: vitamin E because of effect on cellular oxidation, and exchange transfusions because of shift in oxygen hemoglobin affinity (adult red blood cells yield oxygen more readily to tissues and retinal vessels than do fetal red blood cells)
10. Hemorrhagic disease of newborn
    a. A hemorrhagic diathesis in newborn infants who are deficient in vitamin-K-dependent factors
    b. Presents as generalized bleeding tendency within first 3 days
    c. Prothrombin time (PT) and partial thromboplastin time (PTT) prolonged
    d. Treatment consists of 1–2 mg vitamin K. Bleeding stops in 6–12 hours. If hemorrhage is life-threatening, fresh plasma or fresh whole blood transfusion (10 ml/kg) produces immediate results
    e. Since disorder can be prevented by administration of vitamin K, it should be given prophylactically to all newborn infants (1 mg IM)

BIBLIOGRAPHY

Evans HE, Glass L: Perinatal Medicine. Hagerstown, Harper and Row, 1976

Hodgman JE, Freedman RI, Levan NE: Neonatal Dermatology. Pediatr Clin North Am, 18:713–756, 1971

Hoekelman RA, et al: Principles of Pediatrics. Health Care of the Young. New York, McGraw-Hill, 1978

Rudolph AM, Barnett HL, Einhorn AH: Pediatrics. New York, Appleton-Century-Crofts, 1977

Schaffer AJ, Avery ME: Diseases of the Newborn. Philadelphia, W. B. Saunders, 1977

Vaughan VC III, McKay RJ, Nelson WE: Nelson Textbook of Pediatrics. Philadelphia, W. B. Saunders, 1975

3

The Infant, Older Child, and Adolescent— Selected Topics

NUTRITION

A. Infant Feeding
1. *Infancy* includes period up to 2 years
2. Begin solid foods in small amounts 4–5 months of age starting with infant cereal b.i.d.
3. Introduce at monthly intervals pureed vegetables, fruits, meats at midday feeding
4. Introduce *new* foods every 3 days to facilitate identification of specific food idiosyncrasy
5. Sterilization of bottles and formula not necessary
6. Formula may be changed to whole undiluted cow's milk at 3–6 months (warn mother that a change in character of stools may occur)
7. Wean baby from breast or bottle at about 6–18 months
8. Institute chopped or table foods when two teeth appear (usually at 8 months)
9. May skip chopped foods entirely and go directly to table foods
10. Avoid fried or greasy foods, nuts, popcorn, chocolate
11. Do not permit nuts or popcorn until age 4–5 years because of danger of aspiration

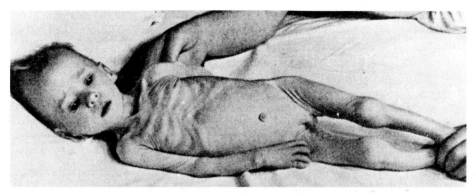

Fig. 13. Marasmic infant aged 10 months. Note loss of subcutaneous fat, most marked over limbs and chest. Facial expression is unhappy and apathetic. (*Hutchison JH: Practical Paediatric Problems. p. 112. A Lloyd-Luke Publication. Chicago, Year Book distributor, 1975*)

12. *In a thriving infant, it is not necessary to calculate daily caloric intake*
13. Discontinue supplementary vitamins and iron at 1 year of age if diet is balanced
14. Warn mother that appetite will fall dramatically at 12–18 months because of normal lag in growth at that time and consequent reduction in daily caloric requirement
15. Parents *must not* coax or force baby to eat
16. Parents *must not* compare food intake of their baby to others—no two infants are the same

B. Infant Colic
   1. Cause unknown
   2. An ill-defined, self-limited symptom complex
   3. Manifest by intermittent abdominal pain characterized by cramping, drawing up legs, screaming
   4. Occurs particularly after evening feeding and may last for several hours
   5. Onset at 2–4 weeks and disappears abruptly at 3–4 months
   6. Must exclude overfeeding, underfeeding, improper feeding, and organic disease
   7. Treatment consists of assurance, instruction in proper feeding (including careful burping), paregoric, phenobarbital, anticholinergic drugs
   8. Parents require continued emotional support and reassurance from physician

C. Failure to Thrive (FTT) (Fig. 13)
   1. Term applies to infants who fail to gain weight. Weight plot is usually below third percentile
   2. Linear growth may also be affected
   3. In extreme cases, head circumference may be affected
   4. Most common cause is *environmental deprivation*
      a. May result from parental ignorance, from want, from neglect

   b. When child is removed from environment (*i.e.*, hospitalized) and fed properly and in adequate amounts, consistent gain in weight becomes immediately apparent
   5. Other causes include renal, central nervous system, cardiac, gastrointestinal disorders
   6. Treatment directed at cause. With environmental deprivation, sometimes necessary to place child in foster home
D. Nutrition in Older Child
   1. Major problem in this age group is overconcern on part of parents. This may result in "problem eater"
   2. "Problem eaters" often result from force-feeding or coaxing, and child learns to use eating habits as attention-getting device
E. Nutrition in Adolescent
   1. Because of social pressures and other problems, many teenagers suffer from improper dietary habits and consequently do not have nutritionally balanced diet
   2. Going without breakfast to be discouraged
   3. Obesity a major problem in this age group
      a. Principal cause is excessive caloric intake
      b. *Treatment:* Generally unsatisfactory. Use of drugs to be condemned. Low-calorie diets successful *only* if patient is committed to losing weight—even then, weight loss most often only temporary
      c. Often, entire family is obese and so problem is compounded
      d. Entire family may need psychologic counseling
   4. Adequacy of diet deserves particular attention in case of vegetarians, health food faddists

GROWTH AND DEVELOPMENT

A. Growth
   1. Length
      a. Extremities grow more rapidly than trunk. At 2 years of age, midpoint is at umbilicus; in adult, midpoint is just below symphysis pubis
      b. Average length at birth is 50 cm (20 inches)
      c. A *crude* estimate of length up to about 10 years of age may be made from following formula: 2 × age in years + 32 = height in inches
   2. Weight
      a. Average birth weight is about 3500 g
      b. Birth weight (*if average*) doubles by 4–5 months and triples by 1 year
      c. A *crude* estimate of weight up to about 10 years of age may be made from following formula: 5 × age in years + 17 = weight in pounds
      d. Greatest increments in growth occur in infancy and in prepubertal period
   3. Head and skull (Fig. 14)
      a. Circumference at birth 32–37 cm

      b. Grows rapidly during infancy with *average* circumference 46 cm at 1 year and 48 cm at 2 years

      c. Cranial sutures do not ossify completely until adult life

      d. Anterior fontanelle usually closes at 3–18 months. Posterior fontanelle usually closes before 2 months

B. Development (Organs and Systems)

  1. *Nervous system:* Superficial reflexes present by 6 months

  2. *Respiratory system:* Rate decreases steadily from up to 50–60/min at birth to 30 by 1 year and 25 by 2 years (adult rate about 18/min)

  3. *Cardiovascular system:* Heart rate falls steadily—130/min at birth, 100/min at 2 years, 90/min at 4 years, 80/min at 6 years, and 70/min at 10 years. Blood pressure increases steadily from neonatal period to age of puberty, approaching maximum at about 14 years in females and about 18 years in males (Figs. 15 and 16)

  4. *Sinuses:* Maxillary and ethmoids present at birth but not aerated for 6 months; sphenoids at 3 years; frontals at 3–9 years

  5. *Special sense organs:* Taste, smell, touch, hearing present at birth. Vision present at birth but not well developed. Tears sparse during early weeks of life. Color perception at 3–5 months; depth perception to some degree at 9 months

  6. *Developmental milestones* (Fig. 17)

  7. *Teeth*

      a. Deciduous teeth are 20 in number

      b. Dentition generally begins at about 6 months. Number of teeth can be crudely estimated by following formula: age in months − 6 = number of teeth for average infant

      c. Teeth appear in following order:

          2 lower middle incisors
          4 upper incisors
          2 lower lateral incisors
          4 molars
          4 cuspids
          4 two-year molars

      d. Adult teeth 32 in number including bicuspids, 6-year, 12-year, and 18-year molars

  8. *Urinary system*

      a. Kidneys immature in neonate and have low urea clearance

      b. Kidneys reach full maturity during second year

  9. *Epiphyseal development* ("Bone age")

      a. Best evaluated by roentgenograms of wrist and hand, but under 2 years of age, roentgenograms of feet and knees also useful

      b. Throughout childhood, epiphyseal development in girls is ahead of that in boys

  10. *Blood*

      a. *Hematocrit:* Newborn = 44–64%; neonate = 35–49%; infant = 30–40%; child = 31–43%; thereafter 40–54% in males and 37–47% in females

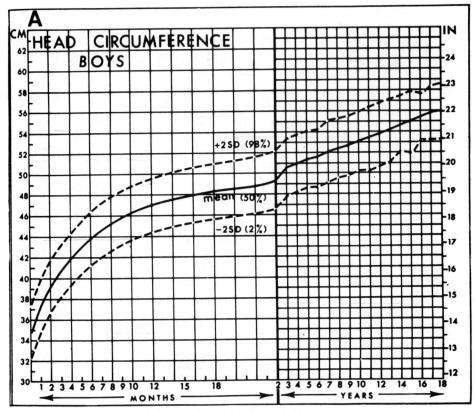

Fig. 14. (A) Composite graph for boys from birth through 18 years.

    b. *Leukocyte count:* Newborn = 9,000–30,000; neonate = 5,000–19,500; infant = 6,000–17,000; thereafter 5,000–10,000. Lymphocytes predominate during infancy

11. *Changes in adolescence*
    a. Sexual maturation related to bone age rather than to chronological age
    b. Girls mature earlier than boys
    c. Adolescent growth spurt in both sexes probably results from androgen production
    d. Pubic hair begins to appear (on the average) at 10–12 years in girls and 12–14 years in boys
    e. Maximum growth spurt occurs about a year before menarche in girls
    f. Menstrual periods at first irregular and may remain so for as long as a year and sometimes longer

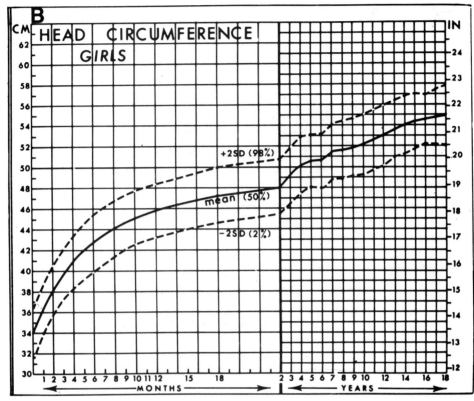

Fig. 14. (B) Composite graph for girls from birth through 18 years.(*Nellhaus G: Head circumference from birth to eighteen years. Practical composite international and interracial graphs. Pediatrics 41:106, 1968*)

12. *Age-related personality characteristics*
    a. Negativistic attitude develops during latter half of second year and reaches peak at 2 years of age, waning thereafter. Referred to as the "terrible twos"
    b. Adolescence characterized by emotional disruption, lack of confidence, self-consciousness, fear of being different, general insecurity, critical attitude toward parents: These tend to wane in late adolescence

PSYCHOSOCIAL PROBLEMS

A. In Infant
   1. Thumb sucking
      a. Normal during infancy

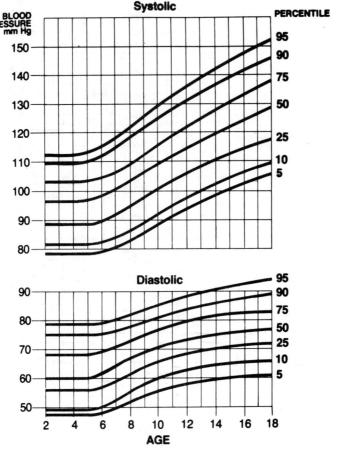

Fig. 15. Percentiles of blood pressure measurement in boys (right arm, seated). (*Blumenthal S et al: Report of the task force on blood pressure control in children. Pediatrics 59:797, 1977*)

   b. Thereafter, occurs with boredom, anxiety, fatigue, during illness, while watching television, and at bedtime
   c. Does not cause dental problems before 4 or 5 years of age. Usually self-correcting at that time
   d. In school-age children is often reflection of deeper emotional problem
2. Resistance to sleep
   a. Some infants resist sleep and demand presence of mother at bedside
   b. Instruct parents to be firm but kind. They should leave room and allow child to cry. After 2–3 nights, situation generally corrects itself
3. Temper tantrums
   a. In infant, are often manifest by *breath-holding* spells
   b. Breath-holding spells characterized by holding breath after inspiration; may

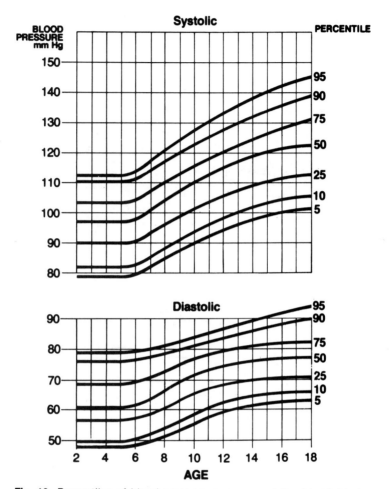

Fig. 16. Percentiles of blood pressure measurement in girls (right arm, seated). (*Blumenthal S et al: Report of the task force on blood pressure control in children. Pediatrics 59:797, 1977*)

terminate in cyanosis, convulsions, loss of consciousness. Recovery usually prompt, and episodes are best ignored. Must be differentiated from epilepsy (if convulsion occurs) and from cardiac disorder (sinus node dysfunction). Epilepsy generally can be excluded by careful history. Cardiac disorder should be suspected if clinical picture is dominated by pallor rather than cyanosis

    c. Breath-holding spells are rare after 3–4 years of age

4. Rocking

    a. Infant may rock rhythmically toward end of first year

    b. Usually ceases spontaneously after few months

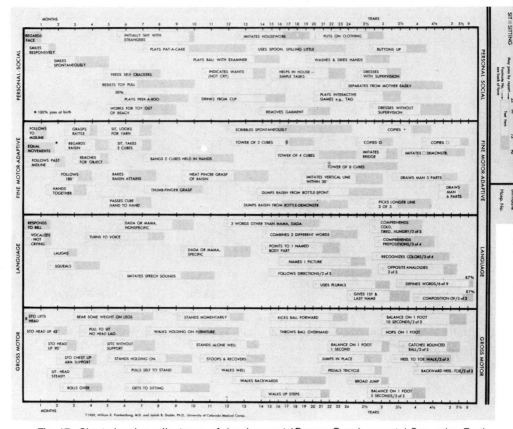

Fig. 17. Chart showing milestones of development (*Denver Developmental Screening Test*).

    5. Head-banging
       a. Bangs head rhythmically against mattress, crib side, or wall
       b. May persist for 2–3 hours at a time
       c. Is benign disorder and disappears before 2–3 years of age
  B. In Toddler and Preschool Child
    1. Sleep disturbances
       a. *Somnambulism* (sleep walking): Common but not serious. If severe may require sedation
       b. *Night terrors:* Differ from nightmares in that sleeping child suddenly sits upright with eyes wide open and screams. Duration only 10 minutes or so following which deep sleep ensues. No recollection of episode next day. Disorder is benign and requires no more than comforting. If severe and frequent, sedation may be helpful. May occur up to about 7 years of age
    2. Encopresis
       a. Defined as fecal soiling after 2–2½ years of age
       b. Common in retarded or emotionally disturbed children

      c. Treatment often requires psychiatric counseling

      d. Organic causes of rectal incontinence must be excluded

C. In School Age Child and Adolescent

  1. Enuresis

     a. Defined as wetting that may be form of constant dribbling during day (diurnal) or wetting while asleep at night (nocturnal)

     b. May be primary (from birth on) or secondary (after 4–5 years of age). However, some normal children may not acquire nighttime bladder control until 6 or 7 years of age

     c. Diagnostic studies include urinalysis only. Intravenous urogram rarely indicated

     d. Usually due to developmental lag, psychoneurotic disorders, tension. Organic basis rare

     e. Treatment varied but consists usually of reward system and drug therapy such as imipramine (Tofranil)

     f. In most cases, cure occurs with or without treatment but disorder may rarely persist into adult life

     g. May be first sign of diabetes mellitus

  2. School phobia

     a. Consists of variety of somatic complaints arising from wish not to attend school

     b. Usually based on fear of something related to school. In young children, may represent a separation anxiety

     c. Symptoms include abdominal pain, headache, vomiting, diarrhea, weakness

     d. Symptoms occur in morning, before school starts, and are limited to school days

     e. Reassurance often corrects situation but school environment should be investigated and in selected cases, psychotherapy indicated

  3. Drug abuse

     a. An increasingly common problem in adolescents

     b. Drugs include wide variety of stimulants, sedatives, hallucinogens

     c. Multiple drugs often taken together

     d. Physician generally sees only "tip of iceberg" (those who suffer severe mental or physical symptoms)

     e. History often not as helpful as one would like since patient may not know name of drug

     f. Should be recognized as *illness* requiring medical, psychologic, and social attention. Punishment and restriction to be avoided

     g. With intravenous administration, hepatitis and endocarditis are potential complications

  4. Anorexia nervosa (Fig. 18)

     a. Uusually in females, usually in late adolescence

     b. Characterized by loss of appetite, severe weight loss, preoccupation with exercise and preparing gourmet foods, amenorrhea, bradycardia, hypothermia, hypotension. Blood carotine levels high

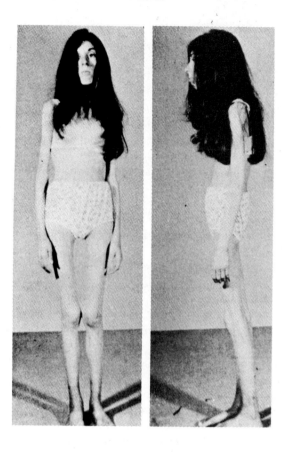

Fig. 18. Advanced anorexia nervosa in a 15-year-old girl. (*Hoekelman RA, Munson SW: In Hoekelman RA (ed): Principles of Pediatrics. Health Care of the Young, p 670. New York, McGraw-Hill, 1978. Used with permission of McGraw-Hill Book Company*)

    c. May reflect psychoneurotic or psychotic disorder

    d. Psychotherapy essential

    e. Carries definite risk to life (although small) and greater risk as far as eventual emotional adjustment is concerned

    f. More prevalent in middle and upper socioeconomic class

5. Attempted suicide

    a. Mainly in adolescents

    b. Represents plea for help, inability to cope, and reflects problem in family or social environment as well as within patient

    c. In about 1 of every 100 attempts, suicide is accomplished

    d. Guns and hanging most common methods of suicide in boys; pills, in girls

    e. Treatment

        1. Early recognition of suicide-prone individuals helpful for prevention. Greatest at risk are "loners" or "outcasts"

        2. For effective prevention, school and home must work together

        3. Proper sex education may be helpful in prevention

        4. Psychiatric evaluation essential

ACCIDENTS

General Considerations
1. Represent the major cause of death in childhood. At least 1 million children per year require medical care and about one-third have some type of permanent disability. Contributing causes are hunger, fatigue, illness or preoccupation of mother, inept baby-sitter, family stresses and tensions, abrupt changes in environment
2. Some children may be accident prone (active, daring, curious)
3. Accidents in childhood include animal bites and injuries; aspiration; automobile, bicycle, minibike, snowmobile accidents; burns; drowning and near drowning; electrical injuries; toy injuries; falls; crib accidents; firearm and firework accidents; playground equipment accidents; wringer injuries; glass door injuries; lawn mower injuries, refrigerator entrapment, skateboard injuries, foreign bodies
4. Treatment should be directed mainly toward *prevention*. Parents and child caretakers *must* be educated in accident prevention. Also, the child, from infancy on, should be educated by the parents. For immediate survey of accident victim, see Figure 19.

POISONINGS

A. General Considerations

Includes ingestion of wide variety of drugs, particularly aspirin, acetaminophin, arsenic (in ant poisons), petroleum distillates, iron, imipramine. Because of extensive list of ingestants, immediate recall of proper management for *all* is impossible. Gastric emptying by lavage or administration of ipecac syrup 15 ml for children followed by a cup of water is standard procedure except for ingestion of petroleum distillates and ingestion of corrosives. If services of a "poison center" are available, they should be utilized for further treatment recommendations. Patient and not poison must be treated first. Attention should be given to need for airway, respiratory assistance, circulatory support, and control of convulsions. All substances that might be useful for analysis should be saved. Activated charcoal one heaping tablespoon in water to be drunk or placed in stomach following gastric emptying—absorbs many drugs (*not* boric acid, alcohols, corrosives, cyanide, ferrous sulfate)

B. Aspirin
1. *Signs and symptoms:* Include vomiting, tachypnea, hyperpyrexia, metabolic acidosis, hypoprothrombinemia
2. *Treatment:* Includes gastric lavage or emesis induction, parenteral glucose and sodium bicarbonate, vitamin K, sponging for fever, and in early severe cases renal dialysis or exchange transfusion

C. Acetaminophen
1. *Signs and symptoms:* Those of severe hepatitis since liver is the target organ

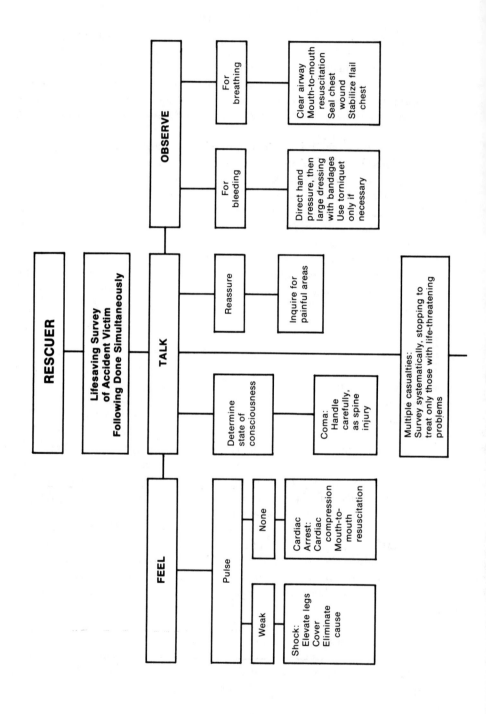

RESCUER

Lifesaving Survey
of Accident Victim
Following Done Simultaneously

OBSERVE

For breathing
- Clear airway
- Mouth-to-mouth resuscitation
- Seal chest wound
- Stabilize flail chest

For bleeding
- Direct hand pressure, then large dressing with bandages
- Use tourniquet only if necessary

TALK

Reassure

Inquire for painful areas

Determine state of consciousness

Coma: Handle carefully, as spine injury

Multiple casualties: Survey systematically, stopping to treat only those with life-threatening problems

FEEL

Pulse

None
- Cardiac Arrest: Cardiac compression Mouth-to-mouth resuscitation

Weak
- Shock: Elevate legs Cover Eliminate cause

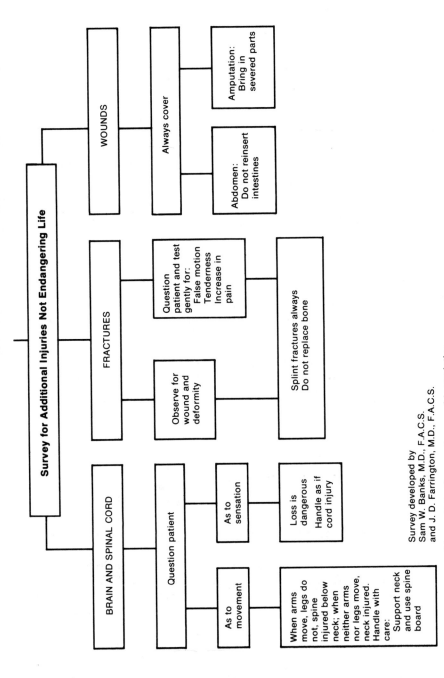

Fig. 19. Schema of immediate survey of an accident victim.

Survey developed by
Sam W. Banks, M.D., F.A.C.S.
and J. D. Farrington, M.D., F.A.C.S.

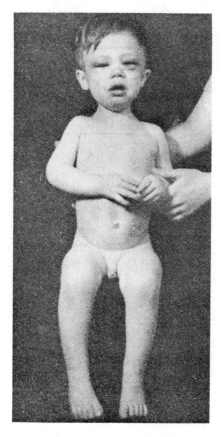

Fig. 20. Battered baby. Note extensive ecchymoses of face and temporal regions and swollen right elbow. (*Hutchison JH: Practical Paediatric Problems, p 556. A Lloyd-Luke Publication. Chicago, Year Book distributor 1975*)

    2. *Treatment:* Gastric emptying, renal dialysis or exchange transfusion in early severe cases, administration of N-acetylcysteine orally or intravenously

D. Arsenic

    1. *Signs and symptoms:* Central nervous and gastroinestinal symptoms, shock, circulatory collapse

    2. *Treatment:* Gastric emptying, administration of BAL and penicillamine

E. Petroleum Distillates

    1. *Signs and symptoms:* Pulmonary insufficiency with pulmonary edema and pneumonia, central nervous system depression

    2. *Treatment: NO* gastric emptying, prevent aspiration, mineral or vegetable oil by mouth, oxygen, antibiotics (controversial), corticosteroids (controversial)

F. Iron

    1. *Signs and symptoms:* Gastrointestinal symptoms, gastrointestinal hemorrhage, shock, liver damage

    2. *Treatment:* Gastric emptying, chelating agents [ethylenediamine tetraacetic acid (EDTA), deferoxamine]. Late follow-up includes gastrointestinal barium studies for strictures; liver function tests

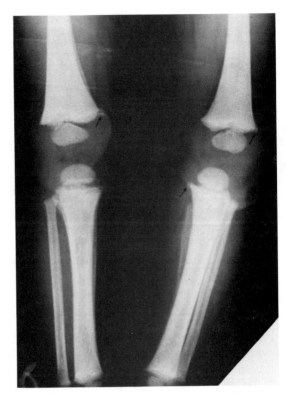

Fig. 21. Roentgenogram of lower extremities of 6-year-old battered child. **Arrows** show metaphyseal corner fractures that are highly suggestive of battered child syndrome. Extensive periosteal reactions are secondary to subperiosteal hemorrhage. (*Courtesy of Dr. H. Kangarloo*)

G. Imipramine
1. *Signs and symptoms:* Coma, convulsions, athetosis,* agitation, visual hallucinations, atropinelike effects, cardiac arrythmias
2. *Treatment:* Intermittent gastric lavage over period of 2–4 days, activated charcoal, intravenous fluids

CHILD ABUSE (BATTERED CHILD SYNDROME)
(Figs. 20, 21)

General Considerations
1. Defined in strict sense as any act of commission or omission on part of parents or caretaker that results in nonaccidental physical or mental injury, or sexual abuse
2. Represents an increasingly common problem that must be differentiated from accidental injury

* See Glossary

TABLE 2 Immunization Schedules
Recommended Schedule for Active Immunization of Normal Infants and Children

2 mo	DTP*	TOPV†
4 mo	DTP	TOPV
6 mo	DTP	‡
1 yr		Tuberculin Test§
15 mo	Measles,‖ Rubella‖	Mumps‖
1½ yr	DTP	TOPV
4-6 yr	DTP	TOPV
14-16 yr	Td#—repeat every 10 years	

* DTP—diphtheria and tetanus toxoids combined with pertussis vaccine.

† TOPV—trivalent oral poliovirus vaccine. This recommendation is suitable for breast-fed as well as bottle-fed infants.

‡ A third dose of TOPV is optional but may be given in areas of high endemicity of poliomyelitis.

§ Frequency of repeated tuberculin tests depends on risk of exposure of the child and on the prevalence of tuberculosis in the population group. For the pediatrician's office or outpatient clinic, an annual or biennial tuberculin test, unless local circumstances clearly indicate otherwise, is appropriate. The initial test should be done at the time of, or preceding, the measles immunization.

‖ May be given at 15 months as measles-rubella or measles-mumps-rubella combined vaccines.

\# Td—combined tetanus and diphtheria toxoids (adult type) for those more than 6 years of age, in contrast to diphtheria and tetanus (DT) toxoids, which contain a larger amount of diphtheria antigen. *Tetanus toxoid at time of injury:* For clean, minor wounds, no booster dose is needed by a fully immunized child unless more than 10 years have elapsed since the last dose. For contaminated wounds, a booster dose should be given if more than 5 years have elapsed since the last dose.

Concentration and Storage of Vaccines

Because the concentration of antigen varies in different products, the manufacturer's package insert should be consulted regarding the volume of individual doses of immunizing agents.

Because biologics are of varying stability, the manufacturer's recommendations for optimal storage conditions (e.g., temperature, light) should be carefully followed. Failure to observe these precautions may significantly reduce the potency and effectiveness of the vaccines.

3. Physical injuries most often include bruises, contusions, welts, hematomas, burns, soft-tissue injuries, fractures, internal injuries
4. Multiple injuries should arouse suspicion
5. Physician must carry out comprehensive workup, inform parents of suspicions, report to designated agency, hospitalize child for protection and evaluation, arrange for multidisciplinary management, provide appropriate treatment for child and family. Placement in foster home may be necessary
6. *Prognosis* for children returned to parents is grave. With repeated abuse, a significant number are killed and about one-third suffer permanent physical damage

TABLE 2 Immunization Schedules (*Continued*)
Primary Immunization for Children
Not Immunized in Early Infancy*

UNDER 6 YEARS OF AGE

First visit	DTP, TOPV, Tuberculin Test
Interval after first visit	
1 mo	Measles,† Mumps, Rubella
2 mo	DTP, TOPV
4 mo	DTP, TOPV‡
10 to 16 mo or preschool	DTP, TOPV
Age 14–16 yr	Td—repeat every 10 yr

6 YEARS OF AGE AND OVER

First visit	Td, TOPV, Tuberculin Test
Interval after first visit	
1 mo	Measles, Mumps, Rubella
2 mo	Td, TOPV
8 to 14 mo	Td, TOPV
Age 14–16 yr	Td—repeat every 10 yr

(Parts a and b: Report of the Committee on Infectious Diseases, 18th ed. Evanston, Ill: American Academy of Pediatrics, 1977)
* Physicians may choose to alter the sequence of these schedules if specific infections are prevalent at the time. For example, measles vaccine might be given on the first visit if an epidemic is underway in the community
† Measles vaccine is routinely given before 15 months of age
‡ Optional

IMMUNIZATIONS

A. General Considerations
   1. Most effective means of preventing infectious disease
   2. Immunizing agents include both bacterial and viral antigens
   3. Bacterial antigens include whole organisms (pertussis), toxoids (tetanus, diphtheria), or attenuated live organisms (BCG). Viral antigens include live attenuated strains (poliomyelitis) or killed vaccines (influenza)
   4. Inactivated vaccines require booster doses. Live vaccines confer immunity more like natural infection—longer duration
   5. Vaccines often combined and administered simultaneously. This does not enhance side effects
   6. Examples of combined vaccines are DPT (diphtheria toxoid, pertussis, tetanus toxoid); DT (diphtheria and tetanus toxoids); TOPV (trivalent oral poliovirus vaccine); measles, mumps, and rubella vaccines; measles and rubella vaccines; Td (tetanus and diphtheria toxoids, adult type)
   7. Combined vaccines given at same time *at different sites* are safe and effective.

These include DPT, DT, or Td plud TOPV; measles, mumps, and rubella virus plus third or fourth dose of TOPV.

8. Single live-virus vaccine injections should be spaced 1 month apart so effects of first injection will not interfere with second, for example, measles virus interferes with yellow fever vaccines

9. Interval between inactivated vaccine (*i.e.,* DPT) and unrelated live-virus vaccine (*i.e.,* measles), should be 2–4 weeks

10. Side effects not uncommon but usually mild. *Local side effects* include mild induration and tenderness but occasionally may be extensive with edema, induration, erythema, tenderness (avoid repeat vaccination with same agent or use fractional doses). *Systemic reactions* include fever, rashes, arthralgia, syncope, allergic reactions. Most subside within 48 hours but with live-virus vaccines, fever and arthralgia may persist for weeks.

11. *Contraindications* include acute febrile illness, immunosuppressive therapy or immunosuppression, recent gammaglobulin, plasma or blood transfusions, pregnancy, leukemia, lymphoma, generalized malignancy, prior allergic reaction to same or related vaccine, simultaneous administration of another single live-virus vaccine unless proved to be effective when given together

B. Routine Immunization for Infants and Young Children

1. Recommended schedule shown in Table 2 can be used for any unimmunized infant or child 2 months–7 years. Also is appropriate for premature and low-birth-weight infants

2. If schedule interrupted, *not* necessary to start series over again

3. Minor afebrile illness such as common cold no indication for interruption of schedule

4. *DPT not to be given after 7 years of age*

5. Severe febrile reaction (over 39°C), somnolence, shock, or convulsions are contraindications for subsequent injections

6. If child has never been immunized, schedule shown in Table 2 is recommended

7. If child has neurologic disorder, may be necessary to avoid all immunizations because there may be adverse febrile and neurologic reactions with risk of further neurologic damage. Each case must be evaluated individually, weighing benefits against potential adverse effects. Adverse effects are less likely to be incriminated in a static neurologic disorder than in a changing one

8. If children with neurologic disorders are vaccinated, antipyretics and phenobarbital may help to reduce reactions

BIBLIOGRAPHY

Blumenthal S et al: Report of task force on blood pressure control in children. Pediatrics 59:797–820, 1977

Hoekleman RA et al: Principles of Pediatrics. Health Care of the Young. New York, McGraw-Hill, 1978

Kempe CH, Helfer RE: Helping the Battered Child and His Family. Philadelphia, J. B. Lippincott, 1972

Kempe CH, Silver HK, O'Brien D: Current Pediatric Diagnosis and Treatment. Los Altos, Lange, 1976

Report of the Committee on Infectious Diseases: American Academy of Pediatrics, Evanston, Ill, 1977

Rudolph AM, Barnett HL, Einhorn WE: Pediatrics. New York, Appleton-Century-Crofts, New York, 1977

Shirkey HC: Pediatric Therapy. Saint Louis, Mosby, 1975

Vaughan VC III, McKay RJ, Nelson WE: Nelson Textbook of Pediatrics. Philadelphia, W. B. Saunders 1975.

Selected Infectious Diseases

DISEASES OF THE RESPIRATORY TRACT

A. Common Cold
1. Etiologic agents
   a. Rhinovirus
   b. Coronavirus
   c. Picornovirus (coxsackie, ECHO viruses)
   d. Myxovirus (parainfluenza, respiratory syncytial virus—latter in adults)
   e. Mycoplasma pneumoniae
2. Manifestations
   a. Incubation period 1–4 days
   b. Nasal congestion, rhinorrhea, sneezing, fever, headache, anorexia, cough
   c. Course usually 5–7 days
   d. May be complicated by sinusitis, otitis media, bronchitis
3. Treatment
      Symptomatic only
B. Bacterial Croup (Epiglottitis)
1. Etiologic agents

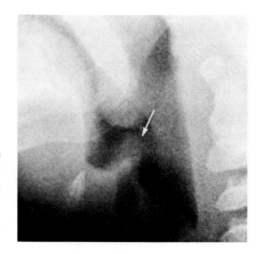

Fig. 22. Bulbous inflammatory swelling of the epiglottis **(arrow)** in *Hemophilus influenzae* epiglottitis. This boy was 16 months old. (*Reproduced with permission from Caffey J et al: Pediatric X-Ray Diagnosis, 7th edition. Copyright © 1978 by Year Book Medical Publishers, Inc., Chicago*)

  a. Hemophilus influenzae B (most common)
  b. Beta-hemolytic streptococcus (rare)
  c. Pneumococcus (rare)
2. Manifestations
  a. Age incidence 2–7 years
  b. Abrupt onset, high fever, difficulty in swallowing, toxic appearance
  c. Rapid progression to respiratory distress, excessive secretions, toxicity, and death, if not treated
  d. Epiglottis is large, swollen, and reddened (great care must be used in visualizing the epiglottis since laryngospasm and sudden death may be precipitated)
3. Treatment
  a. An emergency that requires immediate hospitalization
  b. In case of doubt, lateral x-ray examination of neck confirms presence of large swollen epiglottis, but this must not delay treatment unduly (Fig. 22)
  c. Airway must be established on emergency basis, either by intubation or tracheostomy, depending on facilities and expertise available
  d. *Antibiotics:* Chloramphenicol and ampicillin initially (chloramphenicol because of increasing incidence of resistance to ampicillin)
4. Prognosis
    Fatal if not quickly and appropriately treated
C. Viral Croup (Laryngitis, Laryngotracheobronchitis)
  1. Etiologic agents
    a. Parainfluenza
    b. Adenovirus
    c. Respiratory syncytial virus
    d. Measles virus
    e. Influenza virus

2. Manifestations
   a. Age incidence 3 months–3 years
   b. Gradual onset
   c. Low-grade fever
   d. Laryngeal stridor that may become progressively worse
   e. Cyanosis a late sign
3. Treatment
   a. Mist
   b. Racemic epinephrine by nebulizer or intermittent positive pressure may be helpful
   c. Antibiotics not indicated
   d. Corticosteroids controversial but probably not helpful
   e. Sedation contraindicated (may depress respiratory center)
   f. Oxygen
   g. In severe cases with asphyxia and cyanosis, intubation or tracheostomy may be necessary
4. Prognosis
   Usually good but may be complicated by pulmonary problems (atelectasis, mediastinal emphysema, pneumothorax, pneumonia)

D. Spasmodic Croup
1. Cause unknown (some deny its existence)
2. Manifestations
   a. Abrupt onset
   b. Barking cough
   c. Stridor only mild or moderate
   d. Systemic symptoms mild or absent
3. Treatment
   Mist
4. Prognosis
   Generally good with complete recovery in 3 days

E. Bronchiolitis
1. An acute, self-limited viral infection of young infants (usually under 2 years of age)
2. Etiologic agents
   a. Mainly respiratory syncytial virus and parainfluenza
   b. Less commonly, influenza virus, adenovirus, rhinovirus
3. Manifestations
   a. Gradual onset with coryza,* cough
   b. Wheezing and chest retractions
   c. Dyspnea and cyanosis in severe cases
   d. Roentgenogram shows flat diaphragm with air-trapping
   e. Difficult to differentiate from asthma

* See Glossary

      f. Leukocyte count and differential usually normal

   4. Treatment

      a. Mist

      b. Oxygen

      c. Use of steroids, antibiotics, bronchodilaters, antihistamines controversial but probably not helpful

   5. Prognosis

      a. Course may be stormy

      b. Most infants survive

      c. Disease may be complicated by pulmonary problems (atelectasis, pneumothorax, mediastinal emphysema, pneumonia)

      d. Heart failure rare

F. Bronchitis

   1. Generally an extension of upper respiratory infection and probably due to same organisms

   2. Usually an acute self-limited disease but may become chronic, particularly in smokers and with air pollution

   3. In chronic type, bacteria rather than viruses may be implicated so antibiotic therapy may be indicated

G. Nonbacterial Pneumonias

   1. Mycoplasma pneumonia

      a. Etiologic agent

         Mycoplasma pneumoniae

      b. Manifestations

         1. Peak age incidence 5–19 years

         2. Insidious onset

         3. Fever, cough, chills, malaise in most patients

         4. Sore throat, nasal congestion, coryza in about half of cases

         5. Physical findings usually not remarkable but rales may be audible

         6. Hemogram usually normal but may show leukocytosis

         7. Abnormalities in roentgenogram are generally out of proportion to physical findings

      c. Diagnosis

         1. Positive cold agglutinin test on convalescent serum greater than 1:52 highly suggestive

         2. Definitive diagnosis established by culturing organism from throat or sputum

      d. Prognosis

         1. Good even if untreated

         2. Complications rare but include myringitis,* pleural effusion

      e. Treatment

         1. Erythromycin or tetracycline

* See Glossary

      2. Symptomatic
2. Viral Pneumonias
  a. Etiologic agents
    1. Influenza virus
    2. Measles virus
    3. Parainfluenza virus
    4. Respiratory syncytial virus
    5. Cytomegalovirus
    6. Varicella virus
    7. Adenovirus
  b. Morbidity and mortality
    1. Depends on age of patient, etiologic agent, condition of patient
    2. Influenza pneumonia, varicella pneumonia have particularly high mortality
    3. Varicella pneumonia, cytomegalovirus pneumonia tend to occur in immunocompromised patient
  c. Treatment
    1. Antibiotics of no help
    2. Symptomatic
3. Bacterial Pneumonias
  a. Etiologic agents
    1. Pneumococcus
    2. Staphylococcus aureus (rare)
    3. Klebsiella pneumoniae (rare)
    4. Hemophilus influenzae (rare)
    5. Streptococcus pyogenes (rare)
  b. Manifestations
    1. Cough, fever, tachypnea, dyspnea
    2. Shallow respirations, grunting, flaring of alae nasae, cyanosis
    3. Leukocytosis with shift to left
    4. Infiltrate and sometimes pleural effusion on roentgenogram
  c. Diagnosis
    1. Confirmed by x-ray examination
    2. Responsible etiologic agent demonstrable by culture of blood or sputum. In selected cases, tracheal aspiration or lung tap may be necessary to obtain material for culture
  d. Treatment
    1. Appropriate antibiotic therapy depending on organism
    2. Supportive therapy
  e. Complications
    1. Empyema, lung abscess, sepsis
    2. Staphylococcal pneumonia runs rapid course and has high mortality; is particularly prevalent under 1 year of age and requires prompt anti-staphylococcal antibiotic therapy

ACUTE INFECTIOUS DISEASES

A. Roseola Infantum (Exanthema Subitum, Sixth Disease, Zahorsky's Disease)
   1. Etiology and epidemiology
      a. Etiologic agent not identified but believed to be a virus or group of viruses
      b. Peak age incidence 6 months–2 years. Extremely rare over 4 years of age
   2. Manifestations
      a. Sudden onset with high fever and/or convulsion
      b. Generally do not appear very ill
      c. Fever usually lasts 3 days
      d. Only positive findings usually are slight injection of pharynx, suboccipital lymphadenopathy
      e. When temperature returns to normal, macular eruption appears and remains usually for less than 24 hours
      f. Leukopenia with relative lymphocytosis most pronounced on day of rash
      g. Rarely have encephalopathy
   3. Treatment
      Symptomatic
   4. Prognosis
      Excellent
B. Rubeola (Measles)
   1. Etiologic agent
      Measles virus
   2. Incubation period
      10–12 days
   3. Manifestations
      a. Fever; lassitude; increasing cough, coryza, and conjunctivitis
      b. Photophobia
      c. Just preceding rash, white spots on buccal mucosa (Koplik's spots)
      d. Confluent maculopapular rash beginning on head and face and progressing downward appears on about fourth day
      e. Rash lasts 7–10 days and then may desquamate
      f. Hemogram shows leukopenia with relative lymphocytosis
   4. Treatment
      a. Symptomatic
      b. Antimicrobial therapy for bacterial complications
   5. Complications
      a. Upper and lower respiratory tract (common)
      b. Encephalitis (rare)
      c. Subacute sclerosing panencephalitis (rare, late) SSPE
   6. Prognosis
      a. Self-limited disease
      b. Encephalitis is most serious complication with high incidence of permanent disability and death

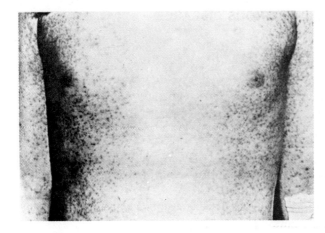

Fig. 23. Atypical measles in a prior recipient of inactivated measles vaccine. (*Eller JJ: In Hoekelman RA et al (eds): Principles of Pediatrics, Health Care of the Young, p 1185. New York, McGraw-Hill, 1978. Used with permission of McGraw-Hill Book Company*)

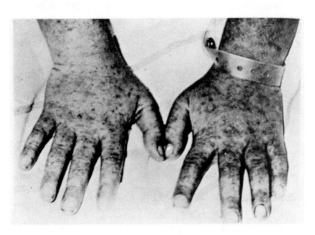

Fig. 24. Atypical measles showing rash on hands in a prior recipient of inactivated measles vaccine. (*Eller JJ: In Hoekelman RA et al (eds): Principles of Pediatrics. Health Care of the Young, p 1186. New York, McGraw-Hill, 1978. Used with permission of McGraw-Hill Book Company*)

    7. Atypical Measles (Figs. 23, 24)
       a. Occurs in children who received killed measles vaccine (identified from history of having received more than single injection)
       b. Characterized by 2–3 day prodrome of fever, malaise followed by petechial, vesicular, urticarial, or maculopapular rash beginning on distal extremities. Pneumonia occurs in almost all cases
  C. Rubella (German Measles)
    1. Etiologic agent
       Rubella virus
    2. Incubation period
       14–21 days
    3. Manifestations
       a. Lymphadenopathy, particularly postauricular and suboccipital

       b. Maculopapular rash beginning on face and descending caudad over a 3-day period

       c. Systemic symptoms minimal

       d. Arthritis not uncommon in adolescent females

   4. Diagnosis

       a. Isolation of virus from throat, blood, urine

       b. Rising antibody titer

D. Varicella (Chickenpox)

   1. Etiology

      Varicella-Zoster virus

   2. Incubation period

      2–3 weeks

   3. Manifestations

       a. Systemic symptoms are mild

       b. Pruritic macules, papules, and vesicles mainly on trunk (Fig. 25)

       c. Lesions become pustular and form crusts

       d. Lesions appear in successive crops over period of up to a week

       e. Lesions may be present in mucosa of mouth and eyes

       f. Low-grade fever may be present as long as lesions continue to appear

   4. Diagnosis

      Clinical criteria usually suffice

   5. Treatment

      Symptomatic

   6. Complications (rare)

       a. Pneumonia

       b. Encephalitis

       c. Encephalopathy and fatty degeneration of liver (Reye's Syndrome)

       d. Glomerulonephritis

       e. Myocarditis

       f. Purpura fulminans

   7. Prognosis

      Generally excellent

E. Scarlet Fever

   1. Etiologic agent

      Group A beta-hemolytic streptococcus

   2. Incubation period

      2–5 days

   3. Manifestations

       a. Pinhead red macules with accentuation in creases (Fig. 26)

       b. Circumoral pallor

       c. Petechial rash on palate (enanthem)

       d. Tonsillar exudate

       e. Cervical adenopathy

       f. Fever

       g. Sore throat

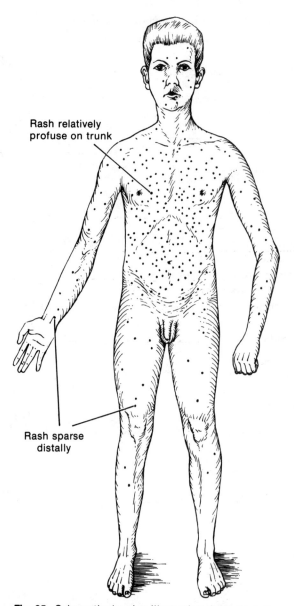

Rash relatively
profuse on trunk

Rash sparse
distally

Fig. 25. Schematic drawing illustrating the typical distribution of the rash of chickenpox. (*Krugman S, Ward R: Infectious Diseases of Children, p 20. Saint Louis, C. V. Mosby, 1964*)

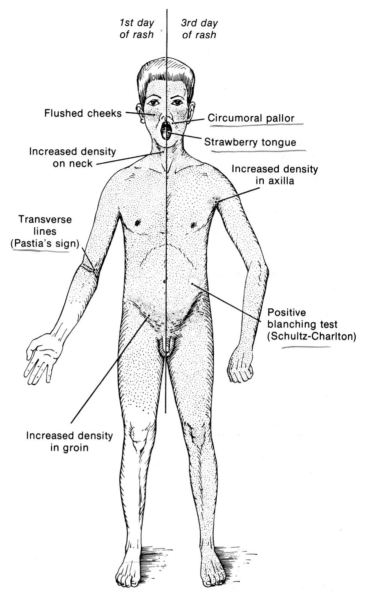

Fig. 26. Schematic drawing illustrating development and distribution of scarlet fever rash. (*Krugman S, Ward R: Infectious Diseases of Children, p 336. Saint Louis, C. V. Mosby, 1964*)

        h. Leukocytosis

        i. Tongue shows white coating with visible papillae ("strawberry tongue") early and "rasberry tongue" later when white coating disappears

        j. Scaling of palms and soles may occur a week or so after onset

    4. Diagnosis

        Clinical criteria plus throat culture

    5. Treatment

        a. Symptomatic

        b. Penicillin × 10 days

    6. Complications

        a. Upper and lower respiratory tract

        b. Sepsis

        c. Rheumatic fever (late)

        d. Glomerulonephritis

    7. Prognosis

        Excellent if recognized and treated early

F. Erythema Infectiosum (Fifth Disease)

    1. Etiologic agent

        Probably a virus, not yet identified

    2. Incubation period

        1–2 weeks

    3. Manifestations

        a. Rash, begins as malar erythema ("slapped-cheek appearance")

        b. Rash becomes maculopapular and finally reticular

        c. Rash spreads to extremities and trunk

        d. Rash lasts 3 days to 5 weeks

        e. Systemic symptoms rare

    4. Diagnosis

        Clinical criteria

    5. Treatment

        None

    6. Complications

        None

    7. Prognosis

        Excellent

G. Mumps (Epidemic Parotitis)

    1. Etiologic agent

        Mumps virus

    2. Incubation period

        2–3 weeks

    3. Manifestations

        a. Enlargement of one or more salivary glands, usually the parotids and usually bilateral (Fig. 27)

        b. May have malaise, low-grade fever, myalgia

        c. Tenderness at angle of jaw common

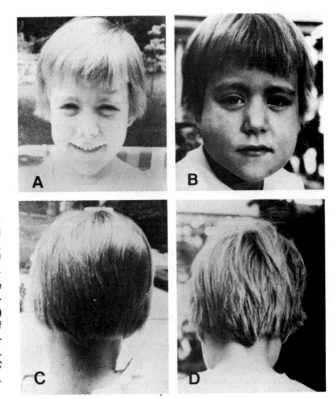

Fig. 27. Mumps. **(A)** Well child. Note sharpness of features and expression. **(B)** Same child. Note expression and change of facial contour caused by bilateral parotid swelling. **(C)** Same well child from rear. Note absence of parotid swelling. **(D)** Bilateral parotid swelling of mumps, often easily appreciated from the rear. (*Grossman M: In Shirkey HC (ed): Pediatric Therapy, p 531. Saint Louis, C. V. Mosby, 1975*)

      d. Orifice of Stenson's duct may be red and swollen
      e. Swelling of salivary glands persists for 1–2 weeks
  4. Diagnosis
      a. Clinical criteria with history of exposure usually suffice
      b. Rising antibody titers
  5. Treatment
      Symptomatic
  6. Complications
      a. Orchitis
      b. Oophoritis
      c. Pancreatitis
      d. Meningoencephalitis
      e. Deafness
      f. Arthritis
      g. Myocarditis
      h. Nephritis
  7. Prognosis
      Fatalities rare

H. Pertussis (Whooping Cough)
   1. Etiologic agent
      a. Bordetella pertussis
      b. *B* parapertussis and adenovirus may cause similar syndrome
   2. Incubation period
         2–3 weeks
   3. Manifestations
      a. Initial *catarrhal* stage* lasting 2 weeks (simulates common cold)
      b. Then *paroxysmal stage* (paroxysms of violent coughing with inspiratory "whoop," often with vomiting. In young infants cough without "whoop" but with apnea and cyanosis). Lasts 2–4 weeks
      c. *Convalescent stage* consists of chronic cough that may continue for months
      d. Leukocytosis with absolute lymphocytosis appears near end of catarrhal stage
   4. Diagnosis
      a. Based on clinical criteria plus history of exposure and peripheral blood count
      b. Identification of organism by culture from nasopharyngeal swab or by fluorescent antibody technique
   5. Treatment
      a. Symptomatic
      b. Erythromycin × 5–10 days
      c. Complications by other bacteria should be treated with appropriate antibiotics
   6. Complications
      a. Pneumonia
      b. Cerebral edema
      c. Cerebral hemorrhage
      d. Bronchiectasis
   7. Prognosis
         Continues to improve but guarded in children under 1 year of age

OTHER DISTINCTIVE INFECTIOUS DISEASES

A. Conjunctivitis
   1. Etiologic agents
      a. Include viruses, bacteria, rickettsiae, and fungi
      b. Wide variety of noninfectious agents
   2. Manifestations
      a. Red eyes
      b. May have blurred vision, photophobia
      c. Mucoid or purulent secretion (Fig. 28)

* See Glossary

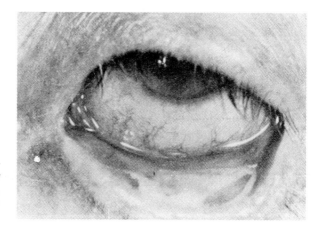

Fig. 28. Pseudomembranous conjunctivitis. (*Furgiuele FP: In Harley RD (ed): Pediatric Ophthalmology, p 267. Philadelphia, W. B. Saunders, 1975*)

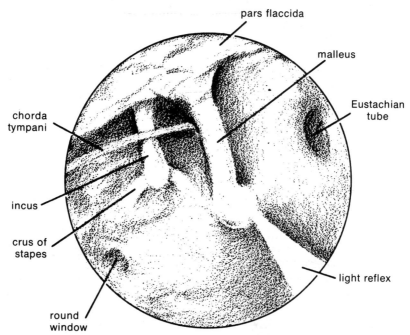

Fig. 29. Diagram of tympanic membrane illustrating the landmarks that should be seen through the normal translucent tympanic membrane. (*Ruben RJ: In Ferguson CF, Kendig EL, Jr (eds): Pediatric Otolaryngology, p 874. Philadelphia, W. B. Saunders, 1972*)

     3. Diagnosis
       a. Gram stain often helpful
       b. Culture
     4. Treatment
       a. Empiric treatment with sulfonamide ophthalmic ointment usually results in improvement
       b. Ophthalmia neonatorum requires vigorous systemic antimicrobial treatment
     5. Prognosis
       Usually subsides within a week
  B. Suppurative Otitis Media
     1. Definition
       Infection of middle ear
     2. Acute purulent otitis media
       a. Epidemiology
          1. Common in young children
          2. Common in children with allergic rhinitis
          3. Usually preceded by upper respiratory infection
          4. More prevalent in winter and spring
       b. Etiologic agents
          1. Usually pneumococcus (40%), Hemophilus influenzae (10–20%), and beta-hemolytic streptococcus (10%)
          2. Viruses (30%)
          3. Rarely Staphylococcus epidermidis (5%)
       c. Signs and Symptoms
          1. Earache
          2. Fever
          3. Nasal congestion
          4. Red, bulging, immobile tympanic membrane, often with fluid level, obliteration of normal landmarks (Fig. 29)
          5. Purulent material in ear canal if tympanic membrane has ruptured
       d. Diagnosis
          1. Typical appearance of tympanic membrane
          2. Etiologic diagnosis established by Gram stain and culture of fluid obtained by tympanocentesis
       e. Complications
          1. Spontaneous rupture of tympanic membrane
          2. Mastoiditis
          3. Meningitis
          4. Brain abscess
       f. Treatment
          1. Antibiotics
             a. Should be given for 10 days
             b. Ampicillin or penicillin plus sulfisoxazole if under 4 years of age
             c. Penicillin if over 4 years of age
             d. Erythromycin plus sulfisoxasole if sensitive to penicillin

      2. Analgesics and antipyretics
        a. Salicylates or acetaminophen
        b. Codeine or demoral if needed for severe pain
      3. Decongestants
          Not of proven value
      4. Myringotomy*
          Indicated in selected cases of extreme pain, persistent high fever, recurrent vomiting
    g. Prognosis
      1. Good if treated adequately
      2. Complications rare
      3. Permanent hearing loss rare

C. Secretory Otitis Media (Serous Otitis, "Glue Ear")
  1. Epidemiology
    a. Due to obstruction of eustachian tube
    b. Commonly associated with allergic rhinitis
  2. Etiologic agents
      Same as for purulent otitis media
  3. Signs and symptoms
    a. Loss of hearing
    b. Feeling of fullness in ear
    c. Crackling sensation in ear
  4. Course and complications
    a. Course variable but usually benign
    b. May be acute, transient, recurrent, or chronic
    c. Permanent middle ear damage or involvement of cochlea with permanent hearing deficit may result
  5. Treatment
    a. Full course of antibiotics as for purulent otitis media
    b. Antihistamines may be of value (controversial)
    c. Decongestants not of proven value
    d. Myringotomy if duration is 2–3 months
    e. Myringotomy with tympanostomy tube placement if duration is more than 3 months

D. Acute Bullous Myringitis
  1. Definition
      Inflammation of tympanic membrane characterized by formation of bullae
  2. Etiologic agents
    a. Same as for purulent otitis media
    b. Occasionally Mycoplasma pneumoniae
  3. Signs and symptoms
      Same as for acute purulent otitis media since this is often associated

---

* See Glossary

    4. Diagnosis

        Visualization of bullae on tympanic membrane

    5. Complications

        Same as for acute purulent otitis media

    6. Treatment

        Same as for acute purulent otitis media

E. Otitis Externa

    1. Definition

        Skin disorder of external auditory canal, meatus, and auricle

    2. Etiologic agents and epidemiology

        a. Usually due to bacteria but may be caused by viruses or fungi

        b. Common in summer months (secondary to swimming) whereas otitis media occurs mainly in winter and spring (secondary to upper respiratory infections)

    3. Manifestations

        a. May be extremely painful, particularly on movement of auricle

        b. Discharge may be present and often has pungent odor

        c. Canal may be swollen and even completely obliterated in severe cases

        d. No systemic symptoms

    4. Diagnosis

        Readily made from clinical manifestations

    5. Treatment

        a. Local cleansing and dry wipes*

        b. Topical instillation of antibiotic–corticosteroid eardrops usually suffices

    6. Prognosis

        Usually improves with local hygiene and treatment

F. Mastoiditis

    1. Definition

        Infection of mastoid antrum complicating suppurative otitis media

    2. Manifestations

        a. Fever

        b. Postauricular swelling, redness, and tenderness

    3. Diagnosis

        a. Clinical manifestations

        b. Roentgenogram

    4. Treatment

        a. Hospitalization

        b. Antimicrobial treatment

        c. Head and neck consultation regarding surgery

    5. Complications

        a. Brain abscess, meningitis

        b. Gradenigo's syndrome (paralysis of abducens nerve)

---

* Parent should be instructed in preparation and use of cotton-tipped toothpicks. Canal should be wiped dry qid (prior to instillation of medication)

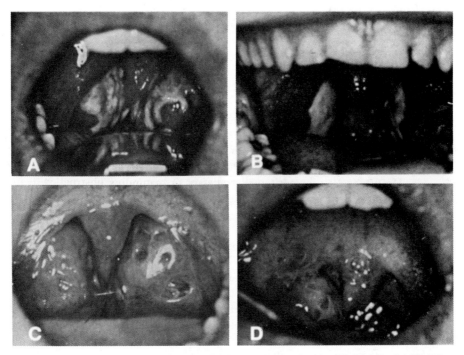

Fig. 30. (A) Tonsillitis associated with infectious mononucleosis. **(B)** Diphtheria. **(C)** Bilateral tonsil and adenoid hypertrophy. **(D)** Unilateral tonsillar hypertrophy. (*Klostermann GF et al: Color Atlas of External Manifestations of Disease, p 209. New York, McGraw-Hill, 1964*)

      c. Bezold's abscess (extension to sternocleidomastoid muscle)

      d. Hearing loss

G. Pharyngitis and Tonsillitis

  1. Definition

     Inflammation of pharynx and tonsils (Fig. 30)

  2. Etiologic Agents and Epidemiology

     a. Usually due to viruses but may be caused by bacteria, fungi, or protozoa

     b. Most frequent bacterial organisms are beta-hemolytic streptococcus, Hemophilus influenzae, and pneumococcus

  3. Manifestations

     a. Bacterial and viral forms may be indistinguishable

     b. Fever, cervical lymphadenopathy, irritability, anorexia, occasionally vomiting, and diarrhea

     c. Pharynx and tonsils are erythematous and swollen

     d. Pharynx and tonsils may be coated with white or yellowish gray exudate (not diagnostic of bacterial infection)

  4. Diagnosis

     Nasopharyngeal culture

5. Complications
    a. Respiratory obstruction secondary to enlarged tonsils (rare)
    b. Peritonsillar abscess
    c. Poststreptococcal glomerulonephritis
    d. Rheumatic fever if streptococcal and untreated
6. Treatment
    a. Symptomatic
    b. Antibiotics if bacterial infection suspected
        1. Penicillin
        2. Erythromycin if sensitive to penicillin
        3. Continue for 10 days if culture positive for streptococcus
    c. Hospitalization for peritonsillar abscess or respiratory obstruction
    d. Tonsillectomy not of proven value for recurrent infections (controversial)
H. Sinusitis
  1. Definition
     Inflammation of one or more paranasal sinuses
  2. Acute form
     a. Etiologic agents and epidemiology
        1. Viral (common)
        2. Bacterial (pneumococcus, Hemophilus influenzae, beta-hemolytic strep-tococcus, and Staphylococcus aureus)
        3. Winter prevalence
        4. More common in allergic individuals
     b. Manifestations
        1. Initial symptoms
           Upper respiratory infection with cough at night
        2. Later symptoms
           a. Fever
           b. Mucopurulent or purulent nasal discharge
           c. Local pain, tenderness over sinuses with or without headache
           d. Epistaxis
           e. Leukocytosis
     c. Diagnosis
        1. Clinical manifestations
        2. Roentgenogram or ultrasound
     d. Complications
        1. Extension to orbit (orbital cellulitis)
        2. Spread from frontal sinus to anterior cranial fossa causing epidural, sub-dural, or brain abscess and/or meningitis
        3. Oral–antral fistula
        4. Hypertrophy of malar bone (maxillary sinusitis) with destruction of bony antrum
        5. Cavernous sinus thrombosis
     e. Treatment
        1. Decongestants
        2. Antihistamines if allergic component present

   3. Antipyretics and analgesics
      a. Acetaminophen or salicylates
      b. Codeine for severe pain
   4. Antibiotics if high fever, severe pain, and leukocytosis
      a. Amoxicillin with trisulfapyrimidines
      b. Erythromycin with trisulfapyrimidines if sensitive to penicillin
   5. Surgery not required in acute case
3. Chronic form
   a. Etiologic agents
      Bacteria most common cause
      a. Same as in acute form
      b. E. Coli, Pseudomonas aeruginosa, anaerobic streptococcus
   b. Manifestations
      Chronic mucopurulent or purulent, foul-smelling nasal discharge
   c. Diagnosis
      Same as in acute form
   d. Complications
      Same as in acute form
   e. Treatment
      1. Same as in acute form
      2. Surgery required if medical therapy fails
I. Thrush (Moniliasis, Oral Candidiasis)
   1. Definition
      Fungal stomatitis caused by Candida albicans (Fig. 31)
   2. Etiologic agents and epidemiology
      a. Candida albicans
      b. Seen in young infants and children with diabetes, malnutrition, and immune deficiency diseases

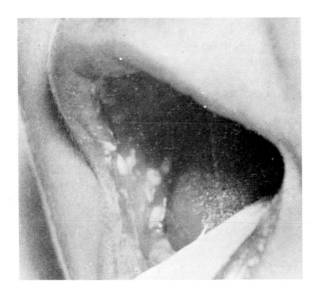

Fig. 31. Oral candidiasis (thrush). (*Jacobs AH: Eruptions in the diaper area. Pediatr Clin North Am 25:209, 1978*)

        c. Not uncommon in normal newborns
    3. Manifestations
        a. Usually no local symptoms
        b. White plaques present on buccal mucosa or palate
        c. Cannot be scraped off without bleeding*
    4. Diagnosis
        a. Clinical
        b. KOH slide preparation made from scrapings of lesion
    5. Complications
        Systemic spread in debilitated patient
    6. Treatment
        a. Nystatin U.S.P.
        b. Amphotericin B for systemic involvement
J. Stomatitis
    1. Definition
        Inflammation of oral mucosa
    2. Herpetic gingivostomatitis
        a. Etiologic agent and epidemiology
            1. Herpes simplex
            2. Common form of stomatitis in children
            3. Most prevalent in children age 1–6 years
        b. Manifestations
            1. Abrupt onset
            2. Fever
            3. Refusal to eat, dysphagia†
            4. Injected gingiva with multiple small ulcers and vesicles on oral mucosa
               (Fig. 32)
        c. Diagnosis
            Clinical signs and symptoms
        d. Complications
            1. Dehydration (uncommon)
            2. Acute herpetic keratonconjunctivitis
            3. Meningoencephalitis (rare)
        e. Treatment
            1. Self-limited course with healing in 5–7 days (10–14 days if severe)
            2. Sympatomatic
                a. Topical 2% viscous lidocaine prior to meals
                b. Analgesics if necessary
            3. Instillation of 5-iodo-2-deoxyuridine (IUDR) for keratoconjunctivitis

---

* Distinguishes thrush from milk deposits
† See Glossary

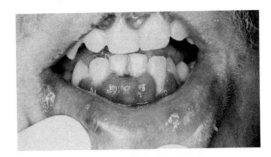

Fig. 32. Primary herpetic gingivostomatitis (*Lynch MA (ed): Barket's Oral Medicine, 7th ed. Philadelphia, J. B. Lippincott, 1977*)

3. Herpangina
    a. Etiologic agent and epidemiology
        1. Coxsackie A virus, occasionally coxsackie B and ECHO viruses are involved
        2. Mainly in summer and fall
        3. Most prevalent in children 1–7 years
    b. Manifestations
        1. Fever
        2. Anorexia, dysphagia
        3. Vomiting, abdominal pain
        4. Anterior oral mucosa less involved
        5. Lesions identical in appearance to herpetic stomatitis
    c. Diagnosis
        By manifestations
    d. Complications
        None
    e. Treatment
        1. Self-limited course (7–10 days)
        2. Symptomatic as in herpetic stomatitis
4. Aphthous Stomatitis
    a. Etiologic agent and epidemiology
        1. Agent unknown (possibly of allergic, traumatic origin)
        2. Occurs in all age groups
    b. Manifestations
        1. No systemic symptoms
        2. Lesions similar in appearance to herpetic stomatitis
    c. Diagnosis
        Clinical manifestations
    d. Complications
        None
    e. Treatment
        Symptomatic as described for herpetic stomatitis

K. Parotitis (Suppurative)
  1. Definition
        Inflammation of parotid gland
  2. Etiologic agent and epidemiology
       a. Most common organism staphylococcus, occasionally streptococcus
       b. Occurs particularly in newborns and debilitated patients
  3. Manifestations
       a. Tender, reddened, swollen parotid gland
       b. Fever may be present
       c. Leukocytosis may be present
  4. Diagnosis
       a. Expression of purulent material from Stensen's duct
       b. Positive Gram stain or culture
  5. Treatment
       a. Hospitalization usually indicated
       b. IV penicillinase-resistant antibiotic initially and then antibiotic coverage according to sensitivities
       c. Drainage of Stensen's duct with 18-gauge needle if obstructed
L. Lymphadenitis
  1. Definition
        Inflammation of lymph nodes
  2. Nonsuppurative
       a. Etiologic agent and epidemiology
          1. Viruses most common organisms
          2. Bacteria less common
          3. Cervical adenitis common with upper respiratory infections
          4. Regional lymphadenitis often secondary to soft-tissue infection
       b. Manifestations
          1. Previous or associated respiratory infection
          2. Soft-tissue infection
          3. Enlarged lymph nodes, usually nontender
       c. Diagnosis
             Signs and symptoms
       d. Treatment
             Treat underlying condition
  3. Suppurative
       a. Etiologic agent and epidemiology
             Beta-hemolytic streptococcus most common. Also pneumococcus, staphylococci, Myobacterium bovis (scrofula), other mycobacteria
       b. Manifestations
             Same as nonsuppurative except lymph nodes are tender, warm, reddened, and may be fluctuant
       c. Diagnosis
          1. Clinical signs and symptoms
          2. Aspirate and culture

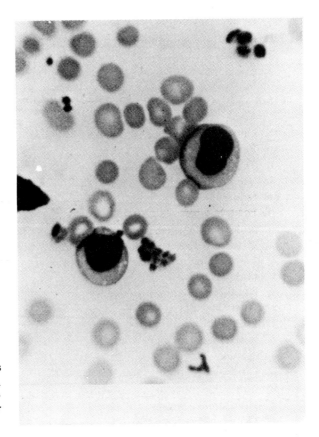

Fig. 33. Typical lymphocytes in infectious mononucleosis. (*Fernbach DJ, Starling KA: Infectious mononucleosis. Pediatr Clin North Am 19:957, 1972*)

      3. Biopsy for suspected mycobacterial infection

   d. Treatment

      1. Penicillin for streptococcus

      2. Penicillinase-resistant antibiotics for staphylococcus

      3. Surgical drainage if fluctuant

      4. Excision and antituberculous drug therapy for mycobacterial infections

M. Infectious Mononucleosis

   1. Definition

      Acute disease of children and young adults manifested by:

      1. Fever, sore throat, and adenopathy

      2. More than 50% lymphocytes and monocytes with at least 10% *atypical* lymphocytes (Downey cells)* in peripheral blood (Fig. 33)

      3. Positive heterophile antibody or monospot test

      4. Abnormal liver function tests

   2. Etiologic agent and epidemiology

     a. Epstein-Barr virus

* See Glossary

     b. In low socioeconomic groups, disease occurs primarily at 2–6 years of age

     c. In high socioeconomic groups, disease usually occurs in teenagers and young adults

     d. Spread probably by oropharyngeal route, but may be result of inoculation by blood transfusion

  3. Manifestations

     a. Fever

     b. Grayish white exudate on tonsils or pharynx (50%)

     c. Palatal petechiae (33%)

     d. Tender lymphadenopathy (includes anterior and posterior cervical chains, but generalized enlargement may occur)

     e. Splenomegaly (50%)

     f. Hepatomegaly (10%), abnormal liver function (nearly 100%), jaundice (4–5%). Abnormal liver function tests usually revert to normal after a few months. No reported instance of chronic liver disease

     g. Maculopapular rash on trunk and proximal extremities (10%) early in course of disease

     h. Neurologic symptoms (1%)

     i. Peripheral blood as described

     j. Leukocyte count 10,000–20,000 but can be as high as 50,000

     k. Positive monospot or heterophile antibody test

  4. Diagnosis

     a. Clinical signs and symptoms

     b. Laboratory tests as described

  5. Complications

     a. Occur in less than 5%

     b. Neurologic complications include Guillain-Barre syndrome,* encephalitis, aseptic meningitis

     c. Splenic rupture

     d. Hemolytic anemia, agranulocytosis, thrombocytopenic purpura

     e. Myocarditis, pericarditis

     f. Airway obstruction from severe tonsillar or pharyngeal edema

  6. Treatment

     a. Symptomatic

     b. Complications

        Glucosteroids for severe tonsillar edema, neurologic sequelae, thrombocytopenic purpura, hemolytic anemia, myocarditis, and pericarditis

N. Urinary Tract Infections

  1. Definition

     Inflammation of any tissue from renal cortex to urethral meatus

  2. Urethritis (male)

     a. Definition

        Inflammation of urethra

* See Glossary

b. Etiologic agents and epidemiology
  1. Neisseria gonorrhoeae
  2. Chlamydia trachomatis
  3. Ureaplasma urealyticum
  4. Miscellaneous organisms
  5. Usually in children over 7 years of age
  6. Almost always secondary to direct sexual contact or handling of genitalia by infected person
c. Manifestations
  1. Dysuria, urinary frequency
  2. Pyuria
  3. Urethral discharge
d. Diagnosis
  1. Clinical signs and symptoms, history
  2. Gram stain of urethral discharge
  3. Early-stream-catch urine is positive, whereas midstream is negative
e. Complications
  1. Proximal extension with cystitis, epididymitis, prostatitis
  2. Sepsis and dissemination
f. Treatment
  1. *Gonorrheal urethritis:* Penicillin G with probenecid, ampicillin with probenecid. Tetracycline or spectinomycin if allergic to penicillin
  2. *Nongonococcal urethritis:* Tetracycline or erythromycin
3. Cystitis
  a. Definition
    Inflammation of urinary bladder
  b. Etiologic agents and epidemiology
    1. E. Coli (50–75%), Aerobacter aerogenes, Proteus species, pseudomonads, enterococci, staphylococci, Candida albicans, miscellaneous
    2. Incidence
      a. Slight male preponderence in newborns. Rarely associated with congenital malformations in this age period
      b. Beyond newborn period, associated congenital malformations are *valves* common
      c. More common in females, in school-age children, and in adolescents
  c. Manifestations
    1. Dysuria, urgency, frequency
    2. Suprapubic pain or tenderness
    3. Urine may be grossly bloody or cloudy
    4. Pyruia, bacteriuria
  d. Diagnosis
    1. Clinical signs and symptoms
    2. Urinalysis
    3. Gram stain and culture of clean-catch specimen
  e. Complications

        1. Pyelonephritis

        2. Sepsis

     f. Treatment

        1. Initial

           Sulfisoxazole or ampicillin

        2. Second and third infections, treat as described previously

        3. Chronically recurrent infections

           Two weeks of antibiotic therapy according to *in vitro* sensitivity followed by sulfonamide for 6 months to 1 year

  4. Pyelonephritis

    a. Definition

        Inflammation of renal parenchyma and renal pelvis

    b. Etiologic agents and epidemiology

        1. E. coli (90%), Klebsiella species, Proteus species, enterococci, Myobacterium tuberculosis, and Candida albicans

        2. Incidence and prevalence unknown

        3. Patients with diabetes, nephrocalcinosis, and sickle cell disease more prone to develop pyelonephritis

        4. May be caused by reflux from infected bladder

    c. Manifestations

        1. Signs and symptoms same as in cystitis plus costovertebral angle tenderness, chills, and fever

        2. Patient may be asymptomatic and present only with pyuria and bacteriuria

    d. Diagnosis

        1. Clinical signs and symptoms

        2. Urinalysis (leukocyte casts) and urine culture

    e. Complications

        1. Chronic pyelonephritis

        2. Perinephric abscess

        3. Chronic renal failure

        4. Hypertension

    f. Treatment

        Intensive antibiotic therapy according to *in vitro* sensitivities. By the intravenous route initially. Should be maintained for a minimum of 2 weeks

O. Periorbital and Orbital Cellulitis

  1. Definition

    Inflammation of tissue in (orbital) and surrounding orbit (periorbital)

  2. Etiologic agents and epidemiology

    a. Staphylococcus aureus, Hemophilus influenzae, and beta-hemolytic streptococcus

    b. Secondary to ethmoid sinusitis

  3. Manifestations

    a. *Systemic:* Chills, fever, malaise, and leukocytosis

      b. *Local:* Tenderness, proptosis,* congestion of eyelids, orbital tissues, and bulbar conjunctiva

   4. Diagnosis
      a. Clinical signs and symptoms
      b. Blood culture

   5. Complications
      a. Cavernous sinus thrombosis
      b. Blindness

   6. Treatment
      a. Moist hot packs
      b. Intensive antibiotic coverage for Staphylococcus, Streptococcus, and H. influenzae

P. Bacterial Meningitis (Beyond 2 Months of Age)
   1. Definition
      Inflammation of meninges accompanied by focal or widespread encephalitis

   2. Etiologic agent and epidemiology
      a. Hemophilus influenzae (25–35%). Mostly in infant age group. Secondary to upper respiratory infection or otitis media
      b. Meningococcus (20%). Secondary to oropharyngeal infection
      c. Pneumococcus (15%). Secondary to upper or lower respiratory infection or otitis media

   3. Manifestations
      a. Fever, vomiting, convulsions, hyperesthesia, pain and resistance on neck flexion, positive Kernig and Brudzinski signs (Figs. 34, 35)
      b. Under 6 months may present only with history of poor feeding, irritability, or lethargy
      c. Headache, photophobia in older children
      d. Petechiae most common with meningococcus infection
      e. Low cerebrospinal fluid (CSF) glucose, high protein, high white cell count with preponderance of neutrophils

   4. Diagnosis
      a. Clinical signs and symptoms
      b. Blood culture
      c. Lumbar puncture for Gram stain and culture
      d. CSF findings as described previously

   5. Complications
      a. Subdural abscess (particularly in hemophilus infections)
      b. Cerebral abscess (particularly in staphylococcal infections)
      c. Hydrocephalus
      d. Ocular nerve palsies, blindness, deafness
      e. Death

   6. Treatment
      Ampicillin and chloramphenicol (for ampicillin-resistant hemophilus and

* See Glossary

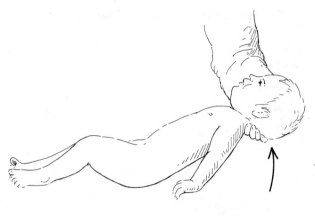

Fig. 34. Illustration of Brudzinski test for meningeal irritation. Patient does not permit passive flexion of neck because of pain.

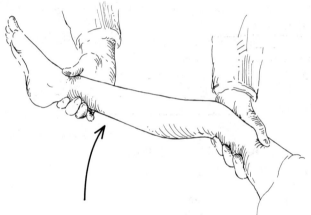

Fig. 35. Illustration of Kernig test for meningeal irritation. Passive extension of flexed knee results in back pain.

other organisms) until cultures establish bacterial sensitivity. Then appropriate antibiotic therapy for 2–3 weeks depending on course and organism
Q. Aseptic Meningitis
 1. Etiologic agents and epidemiology
   Due to wide variety of viruses including enteroviruses, adenoviruses, arboviruses, mumps virus, varicella-zoster virus, lymphocytic choriomeningitis virus
 2. Manifestations
   a. As with bacterial meningitis but usually not as severe
   b. CSF glucose usually normal, protein may be elevated, white cells generally less than 100–200/cu mm with predominance of lymphocytes
 3. Diagnosis
   a. Clinical signs and symptoms
   b. Nasopharyngeal, stool, and CSF cultures for viruses

4. Course
   Usually self-limited
5. Treatment
   Symptomatic

R. Encephalitis
   1. Definition
      Inflammation of brain
   2. Etiologic agents and epidemiology
      a. Viral (most common)
         Transmitted mainly by arthropod bites
      b. Fungal
      c. Bacterial
      d. Protozoal
      e. *Postvaccination:* Acute demyelinating disorder usually after smallpox or rabies vaccination
      f. *Post infectious (secondary encephalitis, allergic encephalitis):* Acute demyelinating process after viral infection (most commonly measles but may occur after chickenpox, rubella)
   3. Manifestations
      a. *Nonspecific:* Gradual or sudden onset fever, headache, lethargy, or coma
      b. *Neurologic:* Specific nerve palsies, ataxia, tremors, and pupillary fixation
      c. *Laboratory:* CSF pleocytosis with up to 1000 leukocytes/cu mm, mainly mononuclear although polymorphonuclear cells can predominate in early phase. CSF sugar usually normal, protein normal or elevated
   4. Diagnosis
      a. Clinical signs and symptoms
      b. Viral titers and cultures
   5. Complications
      a. Secondary bacterial infection of other organs
      b. Residual neurologic defects
   6. Treatment
      Supportive care: Maintaining open airway, fluid and electrolyte balance, adequate nutrition, prevention of bed sores, and prevention of secondary infection

S. Osteomyelitis
   1. Definition
      Inflammation of bone involving cortex, marrow, periosteum, and cancellous tissue
   2. Etiologic agents and epidemiology
      a. Staphylococcus (70–90%)
      b. Streptococcus (next most common)
      c. Salmonella (in sickle cell disease)
      d. Pseudomonas aeruginosa (usually secondary to penetrating wound)
      e. Hematogenous or from infected contiguous structures or from trauma (penetrating wound or fracture)

3. Manifestations
   a. *Local:* Pain, tenderness, erythema, warmth, swelling and reduced joint motion
   b. *Systemic:* Fever, malaise, and tachycardia
   c. *Laboratory:* Leukocytosis with shift to left, elevated erythrocyte sedimentation rate
   d. Radiography (Fig. 36)
      1. Negative until second week of disease
      2. Earliest bone change is radiolucency of affected bone
      3. Bony destruction usually seen around 12th day
      4. Bone scan positive before roentgenographic changes become evident
4. Diagnosis
   a. Clinical signs and symptoms
   b. Laboratory data
   c. Bone scan
   d. Roentgenogram
   e. Bone aspiration and culture
   f. Blood culture
5. Complications
   a. Multiple metastatic foci
   b. Extension into epiphysis and/or joint space
   c. Shortening of affected bone
   d. Chronic osteomyelitis
6. Treatment
   a. Hospitalization
   b. Debridement of skin infection if present
   c. Penicillinase-resistant penicillin for 4–6 weeks. Oral therapy may be instituted after systemic symptoms subside
   d. Ampicillin or chloramphenicol if patient has sickle cell disease
   e. Surgical saucerization* if no response to antibiotic therapy in 48–72 hours
T. Septic Arthritis
   1. Definition
      Invasion of synovial membrane by microorganisms, usually with extension into joint space
   2. Etiologic agents and epidemiology
      a. Staphylococci (40–50% up to 15 years of age, then 15%)
      b. Streptococci (15% under 2 years of age, 25% up to 15 years, then 5%)
      c. Pneumococcus (10% under 15 years, rare over 15)
      d. Hemophilus (30% under 2 years, rare over 2)
      e. Neisseria gonorrhoeae (75% of all cases over 15 years)
      f. Disease caused by hematogenous seeding
      g. Less common causes include penetrating wounds, extension from adjacent osteomyelitis, cellulitis

* See Glossary

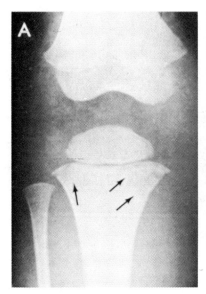

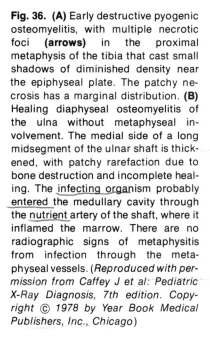

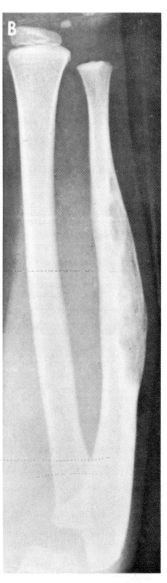

Fig. 36. (A) Early destructive pyogenic osteomyelitis, with multiple necrotic foci **(arrows)** in the proximal metaphysis of the tibia that cast small shadows of diminished density near the epiphyseal plate. The patchy necrosis has a marginal distribution. **(B)** Healing diaphyseal osteomyelitis of the ulna without metaphyseal involvement. The medial side of a long midsegment of the ulnar shaft is thickened, with patchy rarefaction due to bone destruction and incomplete healing. The infecting organism probably entered the medullary cavity through the nutrient artery of the shaft, where it inflamed the marrow. There are no radiographic signs of metaphysitis from infection through the metaphyseal vessels. (*Reproduced with permission from Caffey J et al: Pediatric X-Ray Diagnosis, 7th edition. Copyright © 1978 by Year Book Medical Publishers, Inc., Chicago*)

3. Manifestations
   a. Fever, pain, swelling, limited range of motion
   b. Large joints affected more often (especially knee and hip)
   c. Usually monarticular, but multiple joints may be involved
   d. Gonococcal arthritis
      1. Fever, chills, headache, anorexia, migratory polyarthralgia or polyarthritis
      2. Can present with monarticular swelling, pain, and tenderness
   e. Elevated leukocyte count with shift to left and elevated erythrocyte sedimentation rate
4. Diagnosis
   a. Clinical signs and symptoms
   b. Aspiration of joint fluid for culture, glucose, and cell count
   c. Gram stain of joint fluid
   d. Complete blood count with sedimentation rate
   e. Blood culture
   f. Roentgenogram of joint to rule out coexisting osteomyelitis
5. Complications
   a. Chronic effusion or arthralgia
   b. Functional impairment of joint
6. Treatment
   a. Hospitalization
   b. Antibiotics
      1. *Newborn period:* Oxacillin or nafcillin and gentamicin for staphylococcus and coliforms until culture results are complete
      2. *Under 2 years:* Ampicillin (for Hemophilus influenzae)
      3. *Above 2 years:* oxacillin or nafcillin
      4. Continue antibiotics for 1 week after defervescence of fever
   c. Surgical drainage if patient not improved. However, hip joint should be drained immediately because of danger of vascular compromise with resultant necrosis of femoral head
U. Tuberculosis
   1. Epidemiology
      a. Still an important cause of morbidity and mortality in United States
      b. Spread by droplet infection
      c. Mycobacterium bovis infection (scrofula) results from ingestion of unpasteurized milk or milk products
   2. Pathogenesis
      a. Lung initially infected with spread to regional lymph nodes (primary complex)
      b. Infection controlled immunologically by small T lymphocytes
      c. Hypersensitivity develops 4–8 weeks later (positive skin test)
      d. In infant, initial infection can be severe because of delay in development of resistance
      e. Secondary infection occurs when host immunologic system is compromised

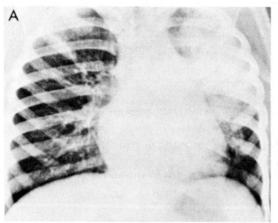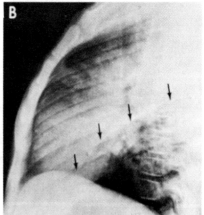

Fig. 37. Large opaque perifocal image (tuberculous pneumonia) in the left upper lobe of a tuberculous girl 8 years of age. **(A)** Frontal and **(B)** lateral projections. Acid-fast bacilli were recovered from the exudate obtained from the left side of the bronchial tree at bronchoscopy. (*Reproduced with permission from Caffey J et al: Pediatric X-Ray Diagnosis, 7th edition. Copyright © 1978 by Year Book Medical Publishers, Inc., Chicago*)

     f. Disease may spread by lymphatics, blood, or by extension and can affect any major organ

3. Manifestations
    a. No symptoms until late in disease
    b. *Pulmonary tuberculosis:* Productive cough, hemoptysis
    c. *Renal tuberculosis:* Pyuria
    d. Roentgenograms show apical or posterior segment homogeneous infiltrate or cavitation (Fig. 37)

4. Diagnosis
    a. History of contact
    b. Positive tuberculin skin test
    c. Sputum or gastric aspirate for acid-fast stain and culture
    d. Chest film

5. Complications
    Disseminated disease

6. Treatment
    a. Who to treat
       1. All patients with active or possibly active disease
       2. Infants, children, and adolescents with positive tuberculin skin test
       3. Recent tuberculin converters
       4. Known tuberculin reactors with diabetes
    b. Drug therapy

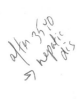

1. Isoniazid (INH) drug of choice. Periodic liver function tests advised because of drug hepatotoxicity
2. Para-aminosalicyclic acid (PAS) enhances effect of INH when used simultaneously
3. Ethambutol
4. Streptomycin
5. Rifampin

  c. INH used alone for 1 year prophylactically in persons with exposure to tuberculosis or with positive skin test

  d. INH used with second drug for 18–24 months in patients with uncomplicated primary disease

  e. Triple drug therapy for tuberculous meningitis or disseminated disease

  f. Skin test all people in close contact with patient

INFECTIOUS DIARRHEAS

A. General Considerations

  1. Definition

    Abnormal frequency and liquidity of stool (more than 20 g/kg/day up to 200 g). Change in bowel movement pattern with loose stools is suspicious of diarrhea

  2. Normal stool pattern

    a. Breast-fed infant up to 8 loose stools per day, which may contain mucus

    b. Infant on cow's milk has less frequent stools that are more solidly formed

  3. Initial evaluation

    a. Establish quantity of diarrhea

    b. Determine if child is able to maintain oral intake

    c. Ascertain presence of associated vomiting

    d. Assess degree of dehydration

      1. *Mild dehydration (5% or less)*: Dry mouth and absence of tears on crying

      2. *Moderate to severe dehydration* (10–20%): Poor skin turgor, sunken eyes, sunken fontanelle (Fig. 38)

    e. Examine stool for blood and leukocytes

    f. Stool culture

    g. Serum electrolytes

    h. Urine osmolality

  4. Treatment

    a. Less than 5% dehydration

      1. Clear fluids by mouth

      2. As diarrhea resolves, add half strength and then full strength low-fat milk; high-protein, low-fat diet

    b. 10% or more dehydration

      1. Hospitalization indicated

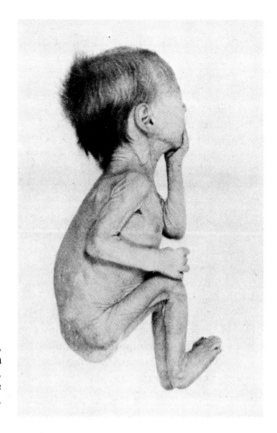

Fig. 38. A female infant, 10 weeks old, showing pronounced wasting after a diarrheal illness. (*Lightwood R, Brimblecombe FSW: Donald Paterson's Sick Children. Diagnosis and Treatment, p 193. Philadelphia, Lippincott, 1963*)

    2. Treat dehydration (see Chap. XII)

    3. When diarrhea resolves, dietary regimen as described previously

B. Viral Diarrhea

    1. Etiologic agents and epidemiology

        a. *Parvoviruslike organisms:* Responsible for major outbreaks of diarrhea in older children and adults

        b. *Rotaviruses:* Major viral source causing sporadic and epidemic outbreaks of enteritis in infants and young children. Present more in temperate zones, highest incidence in winter

        c. *Adenoviruses:* Cause mainly nosocomial infections

        d. Coronaviruslike organisms, minireoviruses, and astroviruses are possible causes

    2. Manifestations

        a. Vomiting, diarrhea, low-grade fever

        b. Mild leukocytosis

        c. Symptoms last 2–8 days

3. Diagnosis

Clinical signs and symptoms

4. Complications

a. Dehydration

b. Electrolyte abnormalities

5. Treatment

As previously described

C. Bacterial Diarrhea

1. Etiologic agents and epidemiology

a. Shigella species

b. Salmonella species

c. Enteropathic *E. coli*

d. Staphylococcal enterotoxin (food poisoning)

e. Campylobacter (common during first 3 years of life)

2. Manifestations

a. Fever, abdominal cramps, watery diarrhea

b. Blood, mucus, leukocytes in stools. Explosive stools in shigella and salmonella infections

c. Prevalence of bands in peripheral blood with shigella infection

d. Staphylococcal enterotoxin infections

   1. Incubation period 3–6 hours

   2. Nausea, *vomiting,* diarrhea

   3. Fever rare

3. Diagnosis

a. Clinical signs and symptoms

b. Stool for leukocytes and culture

c. Blood culture

4. Complications

a. Dehydration

b. Electrolyte imbalance

5. Treatment

a. As previously described

b. Antibiotics

   1. Shigella: Ampicillin. Chloramphenicol for cases not sensitive to ampicillin

   2. Salmonella, E. coli, and staphylococcal infections: Antibiotics not indicated

   3. Campylobacter: Erythromycin may be of value

D. Parasitic Diarrhea

Etiologic agents and epidemiology

a. Entamoeba histolytica (see under Amebiasis)

b. Giardia lamblia (most prevalent in 5–10-year age group)

c. Balantidium coli (rare in United States, common in Mexico and Puerto Rico)

d. Trichuris trichiura (see under Trichurasis)

BIBLIOGRAPHY

Bierman CW, Furakawa CT: Medical management of serous otitis media. Pediatrics 61:768–774, 1978

Gellis SS, Kagan BM: Current Pediatric Therapy. Philadelphia, W. B. Saunders, 1978

Hoekelman RA et al: Principles of Pediatrics, Health Care of the Young. New York, McGraw-Hill, 1978

Hoeprich PD: Infectious Diseases. A Modern Treatise of Infectious Processes. Hagerstown, Harper and Row, 1977

Kagan BM: Antimicrobial Therapy. Philadelphia, W. B. Saunders, 1970

Karmali MA, Fleming PC: Campylobacter enteritis in children. J. Pediatr 94:527–533, 1979

Olson AL et al: Prevention and therapy of serous otitis media by oral decongestant: A double-blind study in pediatric practice. Pediatrics 61:697–684, 1978

Pai CH et al: Campylobacter gastroenteritis in children. J Pediatr 94:589–591, 1979

Report of the Committee on Infectious Diseases: American Academy of Pediatrics, 1977

Rudolph AM, Barnett HL, Einhorn AH: Pediatrics. New York, Appleton-Century-Crofts, 1977

Vaughan VC, McKay RJ, Nelson WE: Textbook of Pediatrics. Philadelphia, W. B. Saunders, 1975

Weinstein L: Infectious disease practice. A Newsletter for the Clinician, 2:1–4, 1978

5

Parasite Infestation

PINWORMS (ENTEROBIASIS)

A. Etiologic Agent and Epidemiology
   1. *Enterobius vermicularis*
   2. Source: Infected humans
   3. Children highly susceptible
   4. Transmission by hand to mouth from perianal region or by inhalation
   5. Eggs remain infective for 2–6 weeks
   6. Practically nonexistent in diaper age
B. Manifestations
   1. Perianal pruritis
   2. Vaginal pruritis
   3. May cause abdominal pain, sleeplessness, anorexia, weight loss
   4. Eosinophilia usually not present
C. Diagnosis
   1. Clinical signs and symptoms
   2. Scotch tape test*

   * See Glossary

D. Complications
   1. Breakdown of perianal skin with secondary infection
   2. Vaginitis or salpingitis in female
E. Treatment
   1. Pyrvinium pamoate, thiabendazole, and pyrantel pamoate are all effective (90% cure rate)
   2. Many times whole family treated because of high reinfection rate
   3. High recurrence rate despite treatment of whole family

ASCARIASIS

A. Etiologic Agent and Epidemiology
   1. *Ascaris lumbricoides*
   2. Resides in small intestine
   3. Larvae hatch from eggs ingested and reach lungs by blood and then mature
   4. Mature larvae travel up airways and then down pharynx
   5. Encountered primarily around Gulf Coast, Appalachians, and Ozarks, although may be seen in northern states
B. Manifestations
   1. Usually asymptomatic
   2. Larvae infestation
      a. Loeffler syndrome (pulmonary infiltrate and peripheral eosinophilia)
      b. Asthma and urticaria
      c. Fever, cough, sometimes hemoptysis
   3. Intestinal infestation (adult worms)
      a. Most prominent symptom is abdominal pain
      b. Nausea, vomiting, anorexia; weight loss and insomnia less common symptoms
C. Diagnosis
   1. Clinical signs and symptoms
   2. Stool for ova and parasites
D. Complications
   1. Intestinal obstruction
   2. Intestinal perforation
   3. Intussusception —
   4. Hemorrhagic pneumonia —
E. Treatment
   1. Piperazine citrate
        80–90% cure rate for one dose; 95% for two doses
   2. Pyrantel pamoate
        90% cure rate

GIARDIASIS

A. Etiologic Agent and Epidemiology
   1. *Giardia lamblia*
   2. Most frequent cause of parasitic diarrhea
   3. Transmission by fecal–oral route
   4. Direct contact transmission occasionally occurs in institutionalized children
   5. Giardia (trophozoite stage) primarily found in small intestine
   6. Gamma-globulin-deficient children particularly susceptible
B. Manifestations
   1. Mild infestation usually asymptomatic
   2. Moderate infestation results in nausea, mild abdominal cramps, distention, flatulence, mild diarrhea
   3. Stools may contain mucus but no blood or white blood cells
   4. Severe infestation can cause vomiting, fever
   5. Patients can present with malabsorption syndrome (foul-smelling stools, flatulence, weight loss)
   6. Infestation may be acute (average duration of symptoms 44 days); subacute (intermittent symptoms lasting months or years); chronic (persists for years)
C. Diagnosis
   1. Clinical signs and symptoms
   2. Identification of cysts in stool
   3. Demonstration of trophozoite in duodenal fluid aspirate (most sensitive test) or small-bowel biopsy
D. Complications
   1. Steatorrhea with malabsorption
   2. Hepatic involvement
   3. Death (rare)
E. Treatment
   1. Infection usually mild and self-limited, thus requiring no treatment
   2. For moderate or severe infections, quinacrine dihydrochloride (Atabrine) results in 95% cure
   3. Second line drug is metronidazole (Flagyl), but is carcinogenic in animals and discretion is advised
   4. For recurrent disease, repeat treatment and investigate patient's environment

AMEBIASIS

A. Definition
   Generally considered to mean infection by *Entamoeba histolytica*
B. Etiologic Agent and Epidemiology
   1. *Entamoeba histolytica*
   2. Man only host
   3. Parasites live in colon and invade mucosa

4. Worldwide distribution with 3–5% infection rate in United States
5. Transmission by fecal–oral route, contaminated food or water
   a. Cysts ingested
   b. In lower small intestine, each cyst disintegrates into several small amebae
   c. Amebae then migrate to large intestine
      1. Expulsion with no pathologic changes or
      2. Proliferation and invasion of mucosa causing ulcerations and clinical symptoms
C. Manifestations
   1. Intestinal disease
      a. Acute
         1. *Mild:* Few shallow ulcerations in cecum and rectosigmoid, fever, abdominal pain, diarrhea, foul-smelling, guaiac-positive stools, leukocytosis
         2. *Severe:* Severe ulceration, fever, diarrhea, grossly bloody stools with mucus, dehydration. Shock may be present
      b. Chronic
         1. *Asymptomatic:* Scattered superficial ulceration of colonic mucosa or just cysts in feces. May have nonspecific abdominal pain, slight diarrhea, or excessive flatulence
         2. *Symptomatic:* Symptoms same as foregoing but can be intermittent, interspersed with constipation. May present as acute or subacute appendicitis, typhlitis (inflammation of cecum), or intestinal obstruction
   2. Extraintestinal disease
      a. Hepatic
         1. Posterior right lobe in 90% of cases
         2. Abscess comprised of degenerated liver cells, fat, inflammatory debris, and amebae
         3. Occurs in 10% of intestinal infestations
         4. Only 50% have prior history of amebic infection and/or diarrhea
         5. More in men than in women
         6. *Signs and symptoms:* Pain radiating to right shoulder, pain right upper abdomen or right lower chest, low-grade fever, weight loss, enlarged liver, jaundice (mild if present)
         7. *Laboratory:* Leukocytosis, abnormal liver function tests, elevated right hemidiaphragm on roentgenogram (Fig. 39)
      b. Pulmonary
         1. Results from direct extension of hepatic abscess through diaphragm
         2. Rarely results from hematogenous or lymphatic spread
         3. Right lower lobe most often involved
         4. *Signs and symptoms:* Hacking cough, fever, chills, right lower thoracic pain, hemoptysis, purulent sputum, signs of pulmonary consolidation and/or pleural effusion
         5. *Laboratory:* Leukocytosis, various stages of lung consolidation on roentgenogram
      c. Cutaneous

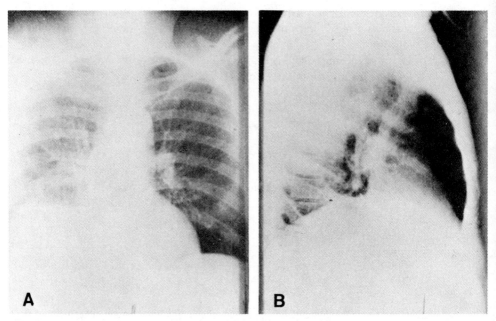

Fig. 39. Posteroanterior **(A)** and right lateral **(B)** chest films showing elevation (fixed by fluoroscopy) of the right hemidiaphragm with compression pneumonitis of the right lower lobe of the lung resulting from amebic abscess in the right lobe of the liver. (*Juniper K: In Hoeprich PD (ed): Infectious Diseases. A Modern Treatise of Infectious Processes, p 578, 1977*)

      1. In 2–3% of invasive amebic disorders
      2. Irregular ulcers in areas adjacent to primary disease (*e.g.,* perianal, abdominal wall, thorax)
      3. Surface of ulcer covered by yellowish gray exudate that when scraped reveals serous or semipurulent fluid containing blood and amebae
      4. Signs and symptoms: Pruritus, dermatitis, urticaria
      5. Mortality high
   d. Cerebral
      1. Rare, caused by hematogenous spread
      2. Signs and symptoms: Similar to those seen in any space-occupying lesion
      3. Usually fatal
D. Diagnosis
  1. Intestinal
    a. Clinical signs and symptoms
    b. Stools for ova and parasites
    c. Intestinal biopsy (sigmoidoscopy)
    d. Indirect hemagglutination test
  2. Hepatic
    a. Confirm intestinal amebic disease
    b. Roentgenogram, ultrasound, CT scan, radioisotopic scan

        c. Indirect hemagglutination test

        d. Aspiration of abscess material if in doubt

    3. Pulmonary

        Same as in hepatic

    4. Cutaneous

        a. Clinical signs and symptoms

        b. Presence of intestinal disease

        c. Examination of ulcer discharge

    5. Cerebral

        Same as in hepatic and pulmonary

E. Complications

    1. Intestinal

        a. Scarring and stricture of colon

        b. Bacterial superinfection

        c. Granulomatous thickening of bowel wall

        d. Hepatic, pulmonary, or cerebral abscess

        e. Cutaneous ulcers

        f. Intestinal obstruction, perforation, hemorrhage, or intussusception

    2. Hepatic

        a. Extension to right lower lobe of lung

        b. Extension to left lower lobe of lung or pericardium

        c. Extension to anterior abdominal wall with fistula formation

        d. Rupture into peritoneal cavity

    3. Pulmonary

        Abscess with rupture into bronchus or pleural cavity

F. Treatment

    1. Intestinal

        a. *Symptomatic:* Metronidazole or paromomycin plus iodoquinol

        b. *Asymptomatic:* Iodoquinol or metronidazole

        c. *Chronic:* Paromomycin plus iodoquinol

    2. Hepatic

        a. Metronidazole

        b. Surgical drainage only if signs and symptoms persist after drug therapy

    3. Pulmonary or cutaneous

        As in hepatic

    4. Cerebral

        a. As in hepatic

        b. Surgical drainage a necessity

TRICHURIASIS

A. Definition

    Infestation by nematodes of the *Trichuris* genus

B. Etiologic Agent and Epidemiology

1. *Trichuris trichiura* (human whipworm)
2. Transmission by fecal–oral route
3. Settle in terminal ileum and cecum
4. Highest incidence of infestation in children 5–15 years
C. Manifestations
   1. Severity of symptoms proportional to number of worms infecting host
   2. *Mild infection:* Asymptomatic
   3. *Moderate infection:* Nonspecific abdominal and lumbar pains, vomiting, diarrhea, or constipation
   4. *Severe infection:* Chronic mucoid or blood-streaked diarrhea, lower quadrant abdominal pain, weight loss, rectal prolapse, microcytic hypochromic anemia
D. Diagnosis
   1. Clinical signs and symptoms not particularly helpful
   2. Stools for ova and parasites
   3. Visualization of adult worm attached to prolapsed rectal mucosa
E. Complications
   1. Severe anemia with heavy infections (500–4000 worms)
   2. Abdominal complications have led to death (extremely rare)
F. Treatment
   Mebendazole

LARVA MIGRANS

A. Cutaneous Larva Migrans (Creeping Eruption)
   1. Definition
      Pruritic, migratory skin eruption evoked by percutaneous invasion and migration of nematode larvae
   2. Etiologic agent and epidemiology
      a. *Ancylostoma braziliense* (hookworm)
      b. Occurs in southeastern United States
      c. Transmission from infected soil to skin
      d. Larvae penetrate skin and migrate within epidermis
   3. Manifestations
      a. Most commonly involve hands, feet, buttocks, genital area
      b. Appearance of lesions diagnostic (serpiginous tracts)
      c. Intense pruritis
   4. Diagnosis
      a. Clinical appearance of lesions
      b. Biopsy of leading edge reveals larva
   5. Complications
      Secondary infection or eczematization as result of scratching
   6. Treatment
      a. Mild infection
         1. Ethyl chloride spray to leading edge

      2. Thiabendazole lotion to lesion
    b. Severe infection
      Thiabendazole
    c. Symptomatic
      1. Aluminum acetate soaks if oozing and crusting are prominent
      2. Topical anesthetic for intense itching

B. Visceral Larva Migrans
  1. Definition
    A syndrome in young children characterized by fever, pulmonary symptoms, hepatomegaly, eosinophilia
  2. Etiologic agent and epidemiology
    a. *Toxocara canis* or *cati*
    b. Infection by ingestion of ova that have been incubating in soil for about 30 days (from dog or cat feces)
    c. Worldwide distribution
    d. Boys infected 2:1 over girls
    e. After ingestion, toxocara hatch in intestine and migrate to portal system with dissemination to rest of body
    f. Granulomas develop in attempt to halt process, but larva sometimes burrows out and continues to migrate
  3. Manifestations
    a. Systemic disease
      1. May be asymptomatic
      2. Fever, cough, wheezing, pulmonary rales, hepatomegaly (Fig. 40)
      3. Central nervous system symptoms include ataxia, convulsions, hemiparesis, coma
      4. Myocarditis (rare)
      5. *Laboratory:* Peripheral eosinophilia (30% or greater), leukocytosis, microcytic hypochromic anemia, elevated IgE
    b. Ocular lesions
      1. Usually late. Rarely occur during systemic disease phase
      2. Lesions consist of posterior pole granuloma, peripheral choroidal lesions, diffuse endophthalmitis with retinal detachment
  4. Diagnosis
    a. Clinical signs and symptoms
    b. Eosinophilia and leukocytosis
    c. High titer of blood group isoagglutinins
    d. Hyperglobulinemia
    e. Precipitating antibody to toxocara antigen in patient's serum (absent in mild infection)
  5. Complications
    a. Chronic liver disease (infrequent)
    b. Ocular lesions
    c. Death (rare)
  6. Treatment

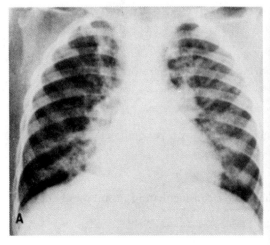

Fig. 40. Chest roentgenograms of a patient with acute visceral larva migrans. There is hyperaeration and bilateral pulmonary infiltration, primarily involving the lower lobes. **(A)** Posteroanterior view. **(B)** Left lateral view. *(Huntley CC: In Hoeprich PD (ed): Infectious Diseases. A Modern Treatise of Infectious Processes, p 643. 1977)*

    a. Diethylcarbamazine (does not prevent ocular disease)
    b. Glucosteroids for treatment of endophthalmitis
    c. Theophylline or aminophylline for wheezing

BIBLIOGRAPHY

Hoeprich PD: Infections Diseases. Hagerstown, Harper and Row, 1977

Report of the Committee on Infectious Diseases, American Academy of Pediatrics, 1977

Rudolph AM, Barnett HL, Einhorn WE: Pediatrics. New York, Appleton-Century-Crofts, 1977

Vaughan VC III, McKay RJ, Nelson WE: Nelson Textbook of Pediatrics. Philadelphia, W. B. Saunders, 1975

Cardiovascular Disorders

INFECTIVE ENDOCARDITIS

A. Definition

Inflammation of endocardium caused by bacteria or fungus

B. Etiologic Agents and Epidemiology

1. Streptococcus viridans (50% of cases)
2. Staphylococcus aureus (33% of cases). More frequent in patients without underlying heart disease
3. Approximately 10% of cases have negative blood culture
4. Staphylococcus epidermidis increasing in frequency as complication of intracardiac surgery
5. Enterococcus (group D streptococcus), rare in children
6. Fungal infection (particularly, Candida albicans) in drug addicts
7. Incidence increasing
8. Disorder occurs as complication of congenital or rheumatic heart disease but can occur in children with normal hearts
9. Rare in infancy
10. Patients with congenital heart lesions that cause high-velocity flow into

chamber or vessels (ventricular septal defect, patent ductus arteriosus, left-sided valvular disease) are at highest risk
11. Surgical or dental procedures implicated in two-thirds of cases
12. Drug addiction
    a. Increasingly frequent in older children and adolescents
    b. *Organisms:* Staphylococcus aureus, Candida albicans, enterococcus, gram-negative bacteria
C. Manifestations
    1. Most patients do not appear particularly ill
    2. Unexplained fever, general malaise, anorexia, weight loss, splenomegaly, murmur of organic heart disease
    3. Embolization rarely occurs with antibiotic therapy
    4. *Osler nodes,* Janeway lesions,* splinter hemorrhages* infrequently seen
    5. *Roth spots* (petechiae with white centers present on mucous membranes) highly suspicious of endocarditis
    6. Increased erythrocyte sedimentation rate, leukocytosis, hematuria, anemia

On Finger or toe
Pard pathogn
of SBE

D. Diagnosis
    1. Clinical manifestations
    2. Blood cultures
    3. Echocardiography may document location of vegetations
E. Complications
    1. Heart failure due to vegetations impairing mitral or aortic valve function
    2. Myocardial abscess or myocarditis
    3. Systemic emboli especially in central nervous system
    4. Mycotic aneurysm, ruptured sinus of valsalva, acquired ventricular septal defect, heart block (all rare)
    5. Death (as high as 25% depending on organism)
F. Treatment
    1. *Streptococcus viridans:* Penicillin
    2. *Staphylococcus aureus and epidermidis:* Oxacillin
    3. *Fungal infections:* Amphotericin
    4. If patient is penicillin sensitive use cephalothin or cephaloridine
    5. Prophylaxis indicated for susceptible individuals (congenital heart disease, drug addicts, history of rheumatic fever) undergoing dental procedures, oral surgical procedures, or any surgery or instrumentation of the body
        a. *For oropharyngeal instrumentation:* Procaine penicillin and crystalline penicillin
        b. For genitourinary instrumentation add streptomycin

INFECTIOUS MYOCARDITIS

A. Definition
    Inflammation of myocardium due to bacteria, rickettsiae, viruses, fungi, protozoa

* See Glossary

B. Etiologic agents and epidemiology
  1. Viruses
     Coxsackie A and B, influenza, ECHO virus, mumps virus, rubella virus most prominent
  2. Bacteria
     Rheumatic fever (streptococcus), meningococcus, diphtheria, gonococcus, pneumococcus
  3. Rickettsiae
     Rickettsia tsutsugamushi (scrub typhus) and R. typhi (epidemic typhus)
  4. Fungi
     Almost all fungi
  5. Protozoa
     Toxoplasma, Trypanosoma cruzi, Leishmania donovani
  6. Patients of all ages afflicted
  7. Worldwide distribution
C. Manifestations
  1. Many asymptomatic
  2. History of preceding upper respiratory infection, nausea, vomiting, myalgia, arthralgia
  3. Malaise, fatigability, dyspnea on exertion, palpitations
  4. Fever, chest pain are important findings
  5. On auscultation, gallops* may be heard due to altered ventricular compliance
  6. Cardiomegaly may or may not be present
  7. Elevated erythrocyte sedimentation rate, myocardial enzymes variable
  8. Electrocardiographic changes also variable
D. Diagnosis
  1. Clinical manifestations
  2. Roentgenogram and electrocardiogram
E. Complications
  1. Congestive heart failure
  2. Arrhythmias
  3. Cardiac arrest
  4. Myocardial fibrosis with chronic cardiomyopathy
F. Treatment
  1. Hospitalization (intensive care unit)
  2. Symptomatic treatment
     a. Decongestive measures for congestive heart failure
     b. Cardiac pacing for heart block
     c. Steroids in selected cases

PERICARDITIS

A. Definition
   Inflammation of pericardium

* See Glossary

B. Pyogenic Pericarditis
  1. Etiologic agent and epidemiology
      a. Staphylococcus aureus (26%), pneumococcus (20%) streptococcus (10%), meningococcus and Hemophilus influenzae
      b. Less common since advent of antibiotics
  2. Manifestations
      a. Fever, tachycardia, chest pain, dyspnea
      b. Heart tones may be decreased, friction rub may be present
      c. May develop neck vein distention, hepatomegaly, pulsus parodoxus* and/or hypotension
      d. Usually leukocytosis (if leukopenia, then poor prognosis)
      e. Abnormal ST segments and T waves on electrocardiogram
  3. Diagnosis
      a. Clinical manifestations
      b. Blood culture, Gram stain, culture of pericardial fluid
      c. Echocardiogram
      d. Electrocardiogram
      e. X-ray examination
  4. Complications
      a. Cardiac tamponade
      b. Sepsis
      c. Constrictive pericarditis
      d. Death (less than 20%)
  5. Treatment
      a. Appropriate antibiotics
      b. Surgical drainage of pericardial sac
C. Tuberculous Pericarditis
  1. Etiologic agent and epidemiology
      a. Mycobacterium tuberculosis
      b. Caused by spread of disease from adjacent lymph nodes
      c. About 25% of all cases occur in children
  2. Manifestations
      Same as for purulent pericarditis
  3. Diagnosis
      a. Same as for purulent pericarditis
      b. Acid-fast stain of pericardial fluid
  4. Complications
      a. Cardiac tamponade (frequent)
      b. Constrictive pericarditis
      c. Death (90%)
  5. Treatment
      a. Antituberculous drugs (see under Tuberculosis)

* See Glossary

  b. Surgical drainage
D. Viral Pericarditis
 1. Etiologic agents
  Coxsackie A and B (especially B), ECHO virus, adenovirus, influenza virus, mumps virus, varicella-zoster virus, vaccinia virus, and possibly others
 2. Manifestations
  Same as for purulent pericarditis
 3. Diagnosis
  a. Clinical manifestations
  b. Electrocardiogram
  c. Echocardiogram
  d. Pericardiocentesis
  e. Viral cultures of nasopharynx, stool, blood, pericardial fluid
 4. Complications
  a. Rare
  b. Cardiac tamponade
 5. Treatment
  a. Symptomatic
  b. Bed rest
  c. Pericardiocentesis* for tamponade
E. Constrictive Pericarditis
 1. Definition
  Thickened pericardium that encases heart and obstructs venous return
 2. Etiologic agents and epidemiology
  a. Predisposing pericardial disease including pericarditis, mediastinal irradiation, neoplastic invasion of pericardium, trauma
  b. Constriction occurs months to years after initial insult
  c. May occur without preceding recognizable disease
 3. Manifestations
  a. Hepatomegaly and ascites are prominent
  b. Distended neck veins
  c. Edema
  d. Minimal respiratory embarrassment
 4. Diagnosis
  a. Auscultation
  b. Cardiac tamponade
  c. X-ray examination including fluoroscopy
  d. Electrocardiogram
  e. Echocardiogram
 5. Treatment
  Radical pericardiectomy

* See Glossary

CONGENITAL HEART DISEASE

A. Patent Ductus Arteriosus (Fig. 41)
  1. Anatomy and hemodynamics
     a. Bridges pulmonary artery and aorta. The anomalous pathway represents persistence of the sixth aortic arch, which maintains its distal connection with the dorsal aorta
     b. Normally closes functionally on first day and anatomically in first year
     c. Usually shunt is from aorta to pulmonary artery (left-to-right shunt) resulting in increased flow to lungs and volume overload of left side of heart
  2. Clinical manifestations
     a. Depend on age of patient and size of shunt
     b. Classic murmur is continuous, maximal at left sternal border in second, third intercostal spaces
     c. During first 6 months of life, diastolic component may be absent because of increased pulmonary vascular resistance with no diastolic pressure gradient between aorta and pulmonary artery
     d. *Small* patent ductus
        Asymptomatic murmur
     e. *Moderate* patent ductus
        1. Poor feeding, irritability, tachypnea, slight retardation of growth, bounding peripheral pulses (due to widened pulse pressure because of systemic run-off from shunt) hyperdynamic precordium with apical thrust (left ventricular enlargement), thrill
        2. Electrocardiogram may show left ventricular hypertrophy. Increased pulmonary vascularity on roentgenogram. Echocardiogram shows increased left-atrial-to-aortic-diameter ratio
     f. *Large* patent ductus
        1. Always symptomatic. Same as with moderate patent ductus plus recurrent pneumonia, rales, heart failure
        2. With congestive heart failure, murmur may become fainter
        3. Electrocardiogram typically shows left ventricular hypertrophy
        4. Chest film shows cardiomegaly with hypervascularity of lung fields
  3. Diagnosis
     a. Clinical manifestations
     b. Electrocardiogram, roentgenogram, echocardiogram
     c. Cardiac catheterization
  4. Complications
     a. Congestive heart failure
     b. Pulmonary vascular disease with pulmonary hypertension. Can progress to irreversible pulmonary vascular obstructive disease and cause shunt reversal (right-to-left). Latter results in cyanosis (Eisenmenger complex*)
     c. Subacute bacterial endocarditis

* See Glossary

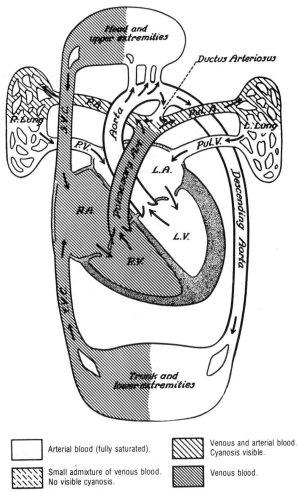

Arterial blood (fully saturated).

Small admixture of venous blood. No visible cyanosis.

Venous and arterial blood. Cyanosis visible.

Venous blood.

Fig. 41. Patent ductus arteriosus. Venous blood returning to the right atrium passes through the tricuspid valve to the right ventricle. It is then ejected through the lungs where it becomes oxygenated and returns to the left atrium. It passes through the mitral valve and enters the left ventricle, from where it is ejected into the aorta. Because of the higher pressure in the aorta than in the pulmonary artery, blood is shunted from the aorta through the ductus arteriosus to the pulmonary artery. This runoff from the systemic circulation increases the work of the left ventricle and causes that chamber to hypertrophy. The increased pulmonary flow results in volume over-load of the left atrium and causes dilatation of that chamber. By the same token, the pulmonary artery becomes dilated. The increased volume in the left side of the heart causes the ascending aorta to dilate.

The continuous flow of blood through the ductus arteriosus during both systole and diastole accounts for the continuous murmur maximal over the pulmonic area. Cyanosis is not observed except in those rare circumstances in which ductal flow is reversed because of high pulmonary vascular resistance (as in pulmonary vascular obstructive disease or in severe pulmonary disease). (*Taussig HB: Congenital Malformations of the Heart, Vol II, Specific Malformations, p 497. Cambridge, MA, Harvard Univ. Press, 1960*)

Eisenmenger

  d. Aneurysm of ductus
  e. Growth failure
  f. Recurrent pneumonia
 5. Treatment
  a. Premature and full term newborn
   1. Restrict fluids
   2. Keep hematocrit above 45% (to prevent heart failure)
   3. Diuretics
   4. Indomethicin
    a. Inhibits prostaglandin synthesis
    b. Permanent closure more likely if therapy started in first 10 days of life
    c. Full response in *very* immature infants less likely
    d. Monitor urine output
    e. *Contraindications:* Bleeding, reduced renal function, disorders of bilirubin metabolism
    f. Should at present be restricted to research protocol
   5. Surgery (if medical management fails)
  b. Infant age group
   1. Decongestive measures for heart failure
    a. Diuretics
    b. Digoxin
   2. Surgery after attempts to stabilize patient
B. Coarctation of Aorta (Fig. 42)
 1. Definition
  Focal constriction of aortic lumen proximal (preductal) or distal (postductal) to origin of ductus arteriosus
 2. Incidence
  a. About 5–10% of congenital heart disease
  b. In infancy, often associated with ventricular septal defect (VSD), patent ductus arteriosus, aortic stenosis
  c. Is most common cardiac abnormality in Turner's syndrome (see Chap. XXI)
  d. Bicuspid aortic valve very common
  e. Mitral valve abnormalities common
 3. Clinical Manifestations
  a. *Infants:* Dyspnea, failure to thrive, overt congestive heart failure
  b. *Older children:* Usually asymptomatic but can have intermittent claudication,* headache, epistaxis
  c. *Physical examination:* Hypertension upper extremities, delayed or absent pulse lower extremities. Grades I–III late systolic ejection murmur at left upper sternal border and in interscapular area
  d. *Chest film:* Aortic constriction with poststenotic dilatation (in older children), sometimes rib notching (Fig. 43) seen mostly after age 3 years (due to collateral intercostal arteries eroding bone), cardiomegaly if heart failure is present

* See Glossary

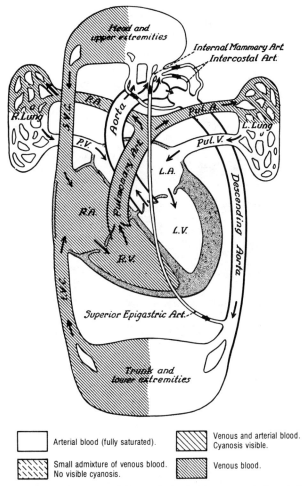

Fig. 42. Coarctation of aorta. The constricted segment of the aorta is most commonly located either proximal to the mouth of the ductus arteriosus (preductal coarctation) or distal to the mouth of the ductus arteriosus (postductal coarctation). In preductal coarctation, some desaturated blood flows from the pulmonary artery through the ductus arteriosus to the low-pressure aorta distal to the coarcted segment. Thus, a mixture of venous and arterial blood supplies the trunk and lower extremities. Under these circumstances, the right ventricle functions as a systemic ventricle and may become hypertrophied. With severe aortic coarctation and a large associated ductus arteriosus, the lower limbs may be cyanotic.

In postductal coarctation, the blood is shunted from the higher pressure aorta through the ductus arteriosus to the pulmonary artery. This results in left ventricular hypertrophy and left atrial dilatation as with isolated patent ductus arteriosus.

If the ductus arteriosus is not patent, the coarctation results in pressure overload of the left ventricle and causes hypertrophy of that chamber.

In all of the preceding circumstances, the pulses are feeble or absent in the lower limbs. However, in the case of preductal coarctation with a large ductal shunt, the lower extremity pulses are sometimes easily palpated, making clinical recognition difficult. (*Taussig HB: Congenital Malformations of the Heart, Vol. II, Specific Malformations, p 799. Cambridge, MA, Harvard Univ. Press, 1960*)

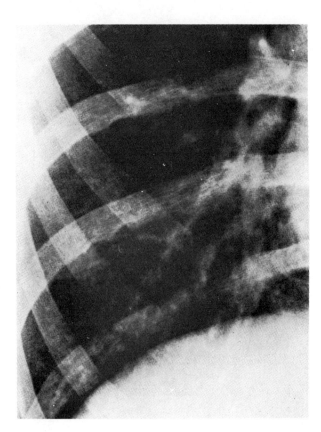

Fig. 43. Notching of the ribs in coarctation of the aorta. (*Taussig HB: Congenital Malformations of the Heart, Vol II, Specific Malformations, p 811. Cambridge, MA, Harvard Univ. Press, 1960*)

    e. *Electrocardiogram:* Variable depending on associated lesions. If isolated, shows left ventricular hypertrophy

4. Diagnosis
    a. Clinical manifestations
    b. Chest film and electrocardiogram
    c. Echocardiogram
    d. Cardiac catheterization

5. Complications
    a. *Infancy:* Early congestive heart failure and death
    b. *Childhood:* Intracranial hemorrhage, rupture of aortic aneurysm, congestive heart failure, bacterial endocarditis

6. Treatment
    a. Infants
        1. Decongestive measures
        2. Cardiac catheterization
        3. Surgery if fails to respond to medical **management**

   b. Children

   Elective surgery at 5–10 years
C. Atrial Septal Defect (Fig. 44)
   1. Definition, anatomy, and hemodynamics
      a. Defect in septum with free communication between atria. Is the result of incomplete partitioning of fetal atrium in region of foramen ovale (secundum type) or of abnormalities in development of endocardial cushions (ostium primum, complete atrioventricular canal, common atrium)
      b. Defect above or at foramen ovale (secundum type) or in lower septum (primum type)
      c. Defect results in left-to-right shunt with volume overload of right ventricle
   2. Incidence and associated lesions
      a. About 5–10% of all congenital heart defects
      b. Associated with Holt–Oram syndrome* and defect in mitral valve (endocardial cushion defect)
      c. Mitral valve prolapse
   3. Manifestations
      a. Secundum type
         1. Often asymptomatic in childhood. Dyspnea, exercise intolerance, congestive heart failure can occur in adult life (rare in infancy or childhood)
         2. Acyanotic, hyperactive parasternal area, grade II–III systolic murmur maximal at upper left sternal border with constant split of second heart sound in pulmonic area. Diastolic murmur often audible over xyphoid area (tricuspid flow murmur)
         3. *Chest film:* Normal or right atrial and right ventricular enlargement with increased pulmonary vasculature
         4. *Electrocardiogram:* Right ventricular hypertrophy
      b. Primum type
         1. Same as for secundum type
         2. Electrocardiogram typically shows *left axis deviation* with right ventricular hypertrophy
   4. Diagnosis
      a. Clinical manifestations
      b. Electrocardiogram and chest film
      c. Echocardiogram
      d. Cardiac catheterization
   5. Complications
      a. Congestive heart failure (late)
      b. Pulmonary vascular obstructive disease with resultant Eisenmenger complex
      c. Bacterial endocarditis notably absent
   6. Treatment
      a. Indications for surgery

* See Glossary

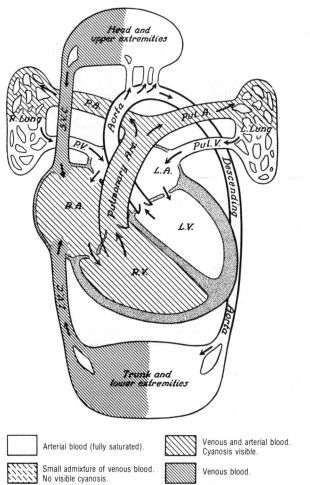

	Arterial blood (fully saturated).		Venous and arterial blood. Cyanosis visible.
	Small admixture of venous blood. No visible cyanosis.		Venous blood.

Fig. 44. Atrial septal defect. Venous blood returned to the right atrium passes through the tricuspid valve to the right ventricle, from where it is pumped into the pulmonary circulation for oxygenation. The oxygenated blood is returned to the left atrium where it passes through the mitral valve to the left ventricle. However, because the pressure in the left atrium is higher than that in the right atrium, some of the oxygenated blood is shunted through the atrial defect into the right atrium and recirculates through the lungs. This volume overload of the right side of the heart results in right atrial enlargment, right ventricular hypertrophy, pulmonary artery dilatation, and hypervascularity of the lung fields. The turbulence of flow in the outflow tract of the right ventricle is the basis for the systolic murmur. With large shunts, relative stenosis of the tricuspid valve may exist and is reflected clinically by a diastolic flow murmur over the tricuspid area.

With the primum type of defect, the mitral valve (and sometimes the tricuspid valve) is defective. The resultant mitral insufficiency can cause varying degrees of associated left atrial enlargement and left ventricular hypertrophy.

In both the secundum and primum types of defects, venous blood does not enter the systemic circulation, so cyanosis is absent. In late adolescence or in adulthood, the development of high pulmonary vascular resistance due to pulmonary vascular obstructive disease may cause the shunt to reverse with resultant cyanosis (Eisenmenger complex). This is not a common complication in the pediatric age group. (*Taussig HB: Congenital Malformations of the Heart, Vol. II, Specific Malformations, p 627. Cambridge, MA, Harvard Univ. Press, 1960*)

Ratio of pulmonary blood flow to systemic blood flow greater than 1.5 : 1 without severe pulmonary vascular obstructive disease

    b. Surgery best done at 2–5 years

D. Ventricular Septal Defect (Fig. 45)

  1. Definition and anatomy

    a. Any defect in ventricular septum that results in communication between ventricles. Is due to failure of the embryonic interventricular foramen to close

    b. Defects classified as small, moderate, large

  2. Incidence and associated lesions

    a. At least 20–25% of all congenital heart disease

    b. May be associated with trisomies 13, 18, and 21

  3. Clinical manifestations

    a. *Small defect:* Asymptomatic throughout life. Murmur may be loud and harsh or may be only grade II in intensity

    b. *Moderate defect:* Congestive heart failure, pneumonia, growth failure, grades IV–VI pansystolic murmur heard best at lower left sternal border

    c. *Large defect:* Same as with moderate defect except that congestive heart failure and pneumonia are more likely to occur. Also, a diastolic murmur (mitral flow murmur) at apex

    d. Chest film may be normal or may show enlarged heart with increased pulmonary vasculature

    e. Electrocardiogram may be normal or show left ventricular, right ventricular, or combined hypertrophy

  4. Diagnosis

    a. Clinical signs and symptoms

    b. Chest film and electrocardiogram

    c. Echocardiogram

    d. Cardiac catheterization

  5. Complications

    a. Pulmonary vascular obstructive disease

      1. In cases of long-standing shunt

      2. Eventually causes shunt reversal with right-to-left shunt (Eisenmenger complex) and patient becomes cyanotic

      3. Poor prognosis

    b. Congestive heart failure

      1. During early months of life pulmonary vascular resistance gradually decreases. This results in increased left-to-right shunting with volume overload of left side of heart and eventual left ventricular failure

      2. Cardiac failure, when it occurs, usually does so at 1–6 months of age

    c. Bacterial endocarditis

  6. Treatment

    a. As high as 50% of small and moderate defects may close spontaneously (usually first 2 years of life)

    b. Initially treat medically (see Ductus Arteriosus, treatment of infant with heart failure)

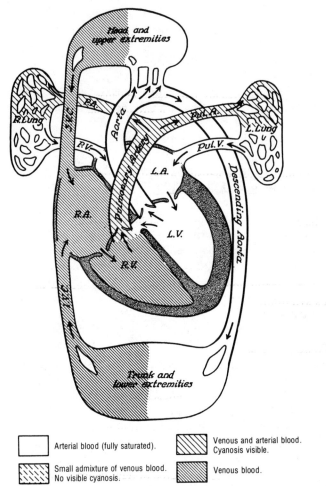

☐ Arterial blood (fully saturated).	▨ Venous and arterial blood. Cyanosis visible.
▧ Small admixture of venous blood. No visible cyanosis.	▨ Venous blood.

Fig. 45 Ventricular septal defect. The defect may be located in either the upper membranous or the lower muscular portion of the septum. In this condition, some of the oxygenated blood in the left ventricle is shunted through the defect into the right ventricle by virtue of the higher pressure in the left ventricle. This causes increased volume of blood in the pulmonary circulation with dilatation of the pulmonary artery and hypervascularity of the lung fields. The increased pulmonary flow results in increased return of oxygenated blood to the left atrium with enlargement of that chamber. The volume overload of the left ventricle causes that chamber also to enlarge and hypertrophy.

Shunting occurs throughout systole and is the basis for the holosystolic murmur. With large shunts, the increased flow of blood across the mitral valve commonly causes a diastolic flow murmur at the apex (relative stenosis of the mitral valve).

With small muscular defects, the opening may close during systole and the systolic murmur may be soft and may occupy only the early portion of systole.

Cyanosis is absent unless pulmonary vascular obstructive disease results in sufficiently high pulmonary vascular resistance to cause the shunt to reverse (Eisenmenger complex). This is not common but is by no means rare. (*Taussig HB: Congenital Malformations of the Heart, Vol. II, Specific Malformations, p 691. Cambridge, MA, Harvard Univ. Press, 1960*)

     c. Patients with high pulmonary artery pressure on first catheterization should be recatheterized at 6- to 9-month intervals

     d. If there is evidence of increasing pulmonary vascular resistance, early surgery is advised

     e. Elective repair at 2–5 years

     f. Surgery not indicated for *small* defects

     g. Patients with Eisenmenger complex are inoperable because correction with high pulmonary vascular resistance imposes a pressure load on the right ventricle and causes right heart failure

E. Valvular Pulmonic Stenosis (Fig. 46)

   1. Definition and anatomy

     a. Any abnormality of pulmonic valve causing a narrowed opening with subsequent increased resistance to flow

     b. Pulmonary valve may be bicuspid with fusion of commissures or tricuspid with thickened leaflets and partial or total fusion of commissures

   2. Incidence and associations

     a. About 5–10% of all congenital heart lesions

     b. May be associated with peculiar facies, short stature, webbed neck, mental retardation, and other somatic defects, but not with chromosomal abnormalities (Noonan's syndrome)

   3. Manifestations

     a. Usually asymptomatic

     b. Dyspnea and exercise intolerance (rare)

     c. Severe stenosis may cause sudden irreversible congestive heart failure in infancy

     d. Grade II–VI, harsh, low-pitched, crescendo-descrescendo systolic murmur (ejection murmur) maximal at second left intercostal interspace with thrill and absence or wide splitting of second heart sound in pulmonic area

     e. Chest film may be normal, but poststenotic dilatation of main pulmonary artery with decreased pulmonary vasculature may be present

     f. Electrocardiogram normal or shows some degree of right ventricular hypertrophy

   4. Diagnosis

     a. Clinical signs and symptoms

     b. Chest film, electrocardiogram

     c. Echocardiogram

     d. Cardiac catheterization

   5. Complications

     a. Congestive heart failure

     b. Bacterial endocarditis

   6. Treatment

     a. Emergency surgery if in congestive heart failure

     b. Asymptomatic patients with *moderate* or *severe* stenosis require elective surgery at 2–5 years of age

     c. Asymptomatic patients with *mild* stenosis require no special attention except for prophylaxis against bacterial endocarditis

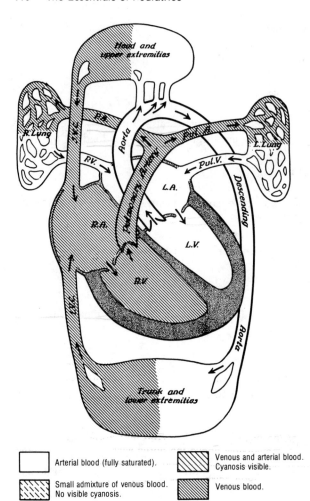

Fig. 46.   Pulmonary stenosis. Regardless of the anatomic location of the obstruction (valvular, infundibular, supravalvular, or peripheral), the hemodynamic effects are essentially the same. Due to impedance of flow from the right ventricle, that chamber hypertrophies and the right atrium also may enlarge.

The murmur is systolic in time and varies in intensity but is *typically* loud and harsh and widely transmitted. Cyanosis is absent. With severe valvular or infundibular obstruction, the second sound in the pulmonic area (pulmonary valve closure sound) is noticeably diminished or absent. (*Taussig HB: Congenital Malformations of the Heart, Vol. II, Specific Malformations, p 389. Cambridge, MA, Harvard Univ. Press, 1960*)

☐ Arterial blood (fully saturated).	Venous and arterial blood. Cyanosis visible.
Small admixture of venous blood. No visible cyanosis.	▨ Venous blood.

F. Aortic Stenosis (Fig. 47)
    1. Definition and anatomy
        a. Any abnormality of aortic valve or adjacent area that causes narrowing of left ventricular outflow tract
        b. Main forms are valvular (majority of cases) and subvalvular
    2. Incidence and associated diseases
        a. Approximately 5% of all congenital heart lesions
        b. Male to female ratio 4 : 1
        c. Occasionally associated with ventricular septal defect, pulmonic stenosis, coarctation of aorta
    3. Manifestations
        a. Acyanotic, grade II–VI crescendo-decrescendo systolic murmur heard best

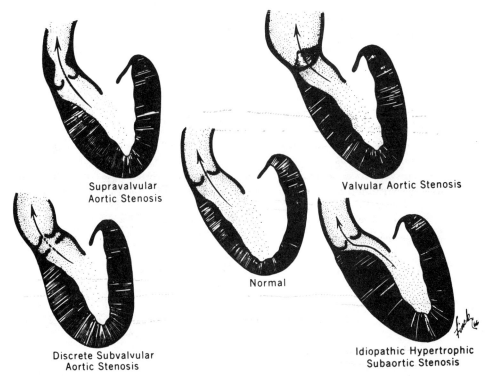

Supravalvular
Aortic Stenosis

Valvular Aortic Stenosis

Normal

Discrete Subvalvular
Aortic Stenosis

Idiopathic Hypertrophic
Subaortic Stenosis

Fig. 47. Diagram illustrating the four basic forms of obstruction to left ventricular outflow. The **central figure** represents the normal left ventricle. In all forms of obstruction, the left ventricular wall is hypertrophied and its cavity is relatively small. The size of the ascending aorta varies, depending primarily on the location of the obstructive lesion. **(Top left)** Aortic supravalvular stenosis. The site of the obstruction is immediately above the aortic valve. **(Top right)** Aortic valvular stenosis. **(Bottom left)** Discrete subvalvular obstruction produced by a fibrous band usually located approximately 1 cm below the aortic valve. **(Bottom right)** Idiopathic hypertrophic subaortic stenosis. (*Braunwald E, Friedman WF: In Watson H (ed): Paediatric Cardiology, p 326. London, Lloyd-Luke, 1968*)

      at first and second right intercostal spaces with transmission to neck, apex, and back

  b. May be asymptomatic or may have mild exertional dyspnea, chest pain, or syncope (ominous signs)

  c. Chest film usually normal. May show poststenotic dilatation of ascending aorta

  d. Electrocardiogram may show left ventricular hypertrophy but is often normal

  e. Cardiac catheterization demonstrates pressure gradient between left ventricle and aorta

4. Diagnosis

  a. Clinical signs and symptoms

    b. Chest film and electrocardiogram

    c. Echocardiogram

    d. Cardiac catheterization

  5. Complications

    a. Bacterial endocarditis

    b. Congestive heart failure

    c. Sudden death

  6. Treatment

    a. Restriction of competitive physical activity in patients with *moderate* and *severe* stenosis

    b. Surgery in patients with symptoms or with severe degree of obstruction

      1. Postoperatively almost all patients left with some degree of stenosis or regurgitation

      2. Most patients eventually require valve replacement

G. Tetralogy of Fallot (Fig. 48)

  1. Definition and anatomy

    a. Is comprised of four anatomic abnormalities: large high ventricular septal defect, right ventricular hypertrophy, pulmonic stenosis, overriding aorta

    b. Pulmonic stenosis may be infundibular, infundibular and valvular, valvular

    c. With associated atrial septal defect, is referred to as pentology of Fallot

    d. Right aortic arch in 25% of cases

  2. Incidence

    About 10% of all congenital heart cases

  3. Manifestations

    a. Usually delayed growth and gross motor development

    b. Acyanotic at birth (cyanosis usually develops during first 6 months)

    c. Dyspnea on feeding, crying, exertion

    d. Squatting

    e. Hypoxic episodes* (cyanotic or "tet" spells). Usually occur in morning and limited mainly to infants

    f. Cyanosis and clubbing of nail beds

    g. Grade II–V systolic murmur along left sternal border. Cause of murmur is the pulmonic stenosis, so the louder the murmur, the milder the pulmonic obstruction

    h. Precordial thrill, polycythemia

    i. Chest film shows normal-sized, boot-shaped heart with decreased pulmonary vasculature

    j. Electrocardiogram shows right axis deviation with right ventricular hypertrophy

  4. Diagnosis

    a. Clinical signs and symptoms

    b. Chest film and electrocardiogram

---

* See Glossary

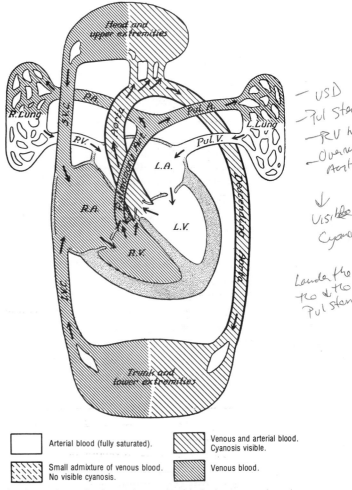

Handwritten margin notes:
- VSD
- Pul Steno
- RV hyper
- Overriding Aorta
- ↓ Visible Cyanosis
- Lander from M to & to Pul Steno

Arterial blood (fully saturated).

Small admixture of venous blood. No visible cyanosis.

Venous and arterial blood. Cyanosis visible.

Venous blood.

Fig. 48. Tetralogy of Fallot. The major hemodynamic determinants in this lesion are pulmonic stenosis and the ventricular septal defect. The latter is uniformly large, and the pulmonic stenosis (whether infundibular or valvular) causes the pressure in the right ventricle to rise. This causes shunting of venous blood from the right ventricle through the ventricular septal defect into the left ventricle. The increased work load of the right ventricle causes that chamber to hypertrophy, and the right atrium enlarges also. Because of decreased flow, the pulmonary artery is small, but the ascending aorta enlarges because of its increased volume. The reduced pulmonary flow results in hypovascularity of the lung fields. Overall heart size is not increased.

The right-to-left shunt through the ventricular septal defect together with the aorta overriding the ventricles results in cyanosis that is usually severe. The systolic murmur reflects the pulmonary stenosis and not the ventricular septal defect because both ventricles have a common ejectile force. The intensity of the murmur is inversely proportional to the degree of right ventricular outflow obstruction—the more severe the stenosis, the softer the murmur. Thus, a progressive diminution in the intensity of the murmur is indicative of increasing severity of disease. (*Taussig HB: Congenital Malformations of the Heart, Vol. II, Specific Malformations, p 15. Cambridge, MA, Harvard Univ. Press, 1960*)

    c. Echocardiogram

    d. Cardiac catheterization

  5. Complications

    a. Cerebral vascular accident* (usually over 2 years of age)

    b. Cerebral abscess (usually over 5 years of age)

    c. Bacterial endocarditis

    d. Hypoxic episodes (usually under 2 years of age)

    e. Congestive heart failure (rare in children)

  6. Treatment

    a. Patients with hematocrits above 65% or with hypoxic spells require surgical relief. Palliative surgery includes Blalock-Taussig operation (right or left subclavian artery to ipsilateral pulmonary artery), Potts anastomosis (left pulmonary artery to descending aorta), Waterston procedure (right pulmonary artery to ascending aorta). All increase flow of desaturated blood to lungs

    b. *Corrective* surgery is preferred and in many centers is done early in infancy

H. Complete Transposition of Great Arteries (d-Transposition, Fig. 49)

  1. Definition and anatomy

    Aorta arises from right ventricle, and pulmonary artery arises from left ventricle so that pulmonary and systemic circuits are in parallel. Some sort of associated shunt is essential for life

  2. Incidence and associated conditions

    a. Approximately 5% of all congenital heart disease

    b. Associated with atrial septal defect or ventricular septal defect, pulmonic stenosis, patent ductus arteriosus

  3. Manifestations

    a. Usually fairly comfortable, cyanotic, large term newborn (more commonly male), progresses to severe cyanosis, dyspnea, poor feeding, congestive failure

    b. Symptoms delayed if large ventricular septal defect present

    c. Physical findings include cyanosis and clubbing, murmurs dependent on associated lesions. Absence of murmur is ominous sign since it indicates only a small shunt

    d. Chest film characteristically shows cardiomegaly with narrow waist and with increased pulmonary vasculature

    e. Electrocardiogram usually shows right ventricular preponderance but may show left

  4. Diagnosis

    a. Clinical manifestations

    b. Chest film and electrocardiogram

    c. Echocardiogram

    d. Cardiac catheterization

  5. Complications

* See Glossary

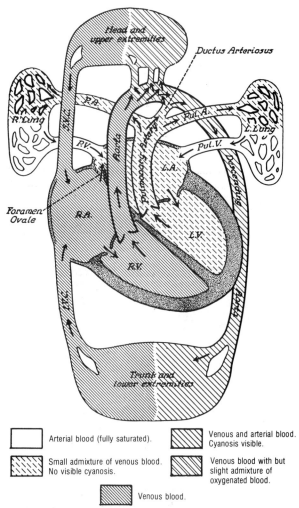

Arterial blood (fully saturated).

Small admixture of venous blood. No visible cyanosis.

Venous blood.

Venous and arterial blood. Cyanosis visible.

Venous blood with but slight admixture of oxygenated blood.

Fig. 49. Transposition of the great arteries. The great arteries are transposed with the aorta arising from the right ventricle and the pulmonary artery arising from the left ventricle. In this condition, the venous blood entering the right atrium passes through the atrioventricular valve to the right ventricle and is ejected into the aorta. It then returns by way of the cavae to the right atrium. In the left side of the heart, blood flows from the left atrium to the left ventricle to the pulmonary artery to the left atrium. The two circuits are thus completely separate and are incompatible with life unless some means for shunting of blood exists (atrial septal defect, ventricular septal defect, or patent ductus arteriosus). The greater the possibility for the circulations to cross, the better the clinical condition of the patient. In fact, atrial septostomy is a palliative procedure aimed at creating or enlarging an atrial septal defect thus permitting the pulmonic and systemic circulations to cross.

Cyanosis is characteristically intense. Auscultatory findings and chamber enlargement are variable depending on associated lesions.

This defect (*dextro* transposition of the great arteries) is not to be confused with congenitally corrected transposition of the great arteries (*levo* transposition). In the latter case, the great arteries arise from the proper ventricle, but the architecture of the two ventricles is transposed, the right ventricular wall being smooth and with a bicuspid atrioventricular valve whereas the left ventricular wall is trabeculated and the atrioventricular valve is tricuspid. The great arteries lie side by side and *appear* to be transposed but are not. Associated lesions are almost invariably present and determine the symptomatology and prognosis. (*Taussig HB: Congenital Malformations of the Heart, Vol. II, Specific Malformations, p 153, Cambridge, MA, Harvard Univ. Press, 1960*)

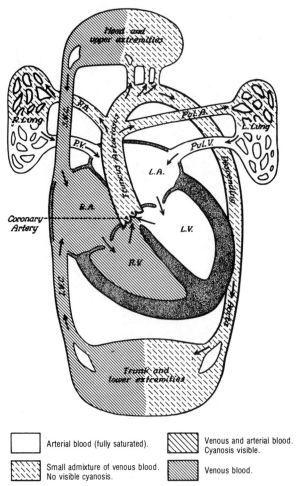

	Arterial blood (fully saturated).		Venous and arterial blood. Cyanosis visible.
	Small admixture of venous blood. No visible cyanosis.		Venous blood.

Fig. 50. Truncus Arteriosus. This lesion is characterized by failure of the fetal truncoconal channel to divide into two independent structures, the aorta and the pulmonary artery. Depending on the degree of maldevelopment, the pulmonary artery may be large, small, or absent. In any event, only one valve exists (the truncal valve). The valve itself is malformed and may have as many as six cusps. Since there is only a single valve, an associated ventricular septal defect is a necessary part of the lesion.

The degree of cyanosis depends on the presence or absence of pulmonary arteries. With large pulmonary flow, visible cyanosis is minimal or may even be absent. If pulmonary arteries are not present and the lungs are dependent entirely on bronchial flow, cyanosis is intense. Auscultatory, electrocardiographic, and roentgenographic features are variable depending on the amount of pulmonary flow. In any event, the second sound in the pulmonic area is usually loud and single, and a diastolic murmur often reflects insufficiency of the truncal valve. (*Taussig HB: Congenital Malformations of the Heart, Vol. II, Specific Malformations, p 289. Cambridge, MA, Harvard Univ. Press, 1960*)

a. Congestive heart failure
b. Cerebral thrombosis
c. Cerebral abscess
d. Pulmonary vascular disease
6. Treatment
a. If untreated, most patients die under 6 months of age
b. Immediate atrial septostomy*
c. Surgery required for all, preferably at about 1 year of age
d. Mustard procedure most favored operation
   1. Redirects systemic blood to left ventricle and displaced pulmonary artery and pulmonary venous blood to right ventricle and aorta by construction of intra-atrial baffle
   2. Operative mortality 5–15%
I. Truncus Arteriosus (Fig. 50)
1. Definition and anatomy
a. Failure of septation of primitive aortopulmonary trunk
b. *Type I:* Common aortic and pulmonary trunk
c. *Type II:* Pulmonary arteries arise from posterior part of trunk
d. *Type III:* Pulmonary arteries arise from lateral portion of trunk
e. *Type IV:* No pulmonary arteries. Lungs supplied by bronchial arteries only
f. All types *must* have a ventricular septal defect
2. Incidence and associated conditions
a. Less than 5% of all congenital heart disease
b. Associated with right aortic arch (common), patent ductus arteriosus, complete interruption of aortic arch, unilateral pulmonary artery atresia, atrial septal defect, partial anomalous venous return
3. Manifestations
a. Mild to severe cyanosis, tachypnea, tachycardia, and poor feeding
b. In type IV, cyanosis is marked
c. Physical findings include cyanosis, prominent peripheral pulses, systolic thrill,* loud ejection click,* pansystolic, diastolic, or continuous murmur maximal at lower left sternal border
d. Chest film shows cardiomegaly with increased or decreased pulmonary vasculature. May see right aortic arch, abnormally high origin of left pulmonary artery, large truncal root, or no main pulmonary artery
J. Hypoplastic Left Heart Syndrome (Fig. 51)
1. Definition and anatomy
a. Underdeveloped, essentially nonfunctioning left ventricle
b. Two types
   1. Marked stenosis or atresia of aortic valve; associated hypoplasia or atresia of mitral valve
   2. Only mitral valve atresia, aortic valve normal

* See Glossary

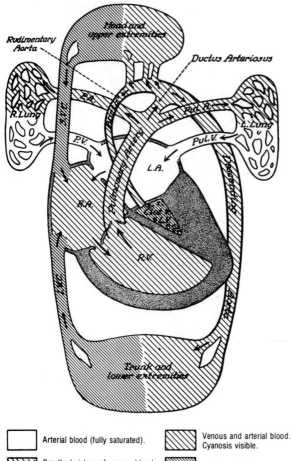

Fig. 51. Hypoplastic left heart syndrome. The left ventricle is underdeveloped and there is marked stenosis or atresia of the aortic and mitral valves. In its most extreme form, blood returning to the left atrium from the pulmonary circuit can only exit through a patent foramen ovale and recirculate through the right atrium and right ventricle. The aorta receives its blood supply by way of the ductus arteriosus. Thus, an interatrial communication and patency of the ductus arteriosus are both necessary for life. (*Taussig HB: Congenital Malformations of the Heart, Vol. II, Specific Malformations, p 261. Cambridge, MA, Harvard Univ. Press, 1960*)

Arterial blood (fully saturated).

Small admixture of venous blood. No visible cyanosis.

Venous and arterial blood. Cyanosis visible.

Venous blood.

2. Incidence and associations

Less than 5% of all congenital heart disease

3. Manifestations

a. Normal at birth (majority)

b. Abrupt onset of cyanosis and respiratory distress (during first week of life)

c. Poor peripheral pulses

d. Progressive downhill course

e. Invariably fatal

f. Grade I–III systolic murmur heard best along left sternal border and over pulmonic area (present in ⅔ of cases)

g. Tachypnea, tachycardia, gallop, rales, hepatomegaly, and occasionally edema

h. Pallor, cyanosis (mild if present at all)

      i. Chest film shows enlarged heart with increased pulmonary flow

      j. Electrocardiogram shows tall peaked P waves, right axis deviation, right ventricular hypertrophy, and absence of left ventricular forces

      k. Echocardiogram fails to demonstrate mitral valve, and aortic root is small or absent

    4. Diagnosis

      a. Clinical signs and symptoms

      b. Chest film and electrocardiogram

      c. Echocardiography and cardiac catheterization

    5. Complications

        Death (100%)

    6. Treatment

        None

K. Total Anomalous Venous Return (Fig. 52)

    1. Definition and anatomy

      a. Drainage of all pulmonary veins to right atrium instead of left

      b. Four common types

        1. Drainage into superior vena cava

        2. Drainage into coronary sinus

        3. Direct connection to right atrium

        4. Drainage into portal vein

    2. Incidence and associated diseases

      a. Less than 1% incidence

      b. *Must* be associated with atrial septal defect to be compatible with life

    3. Manifestations

      a. If pulmonary venous obstruction present, cyanosis and tachypnea at birth with progressive downhill course

      b. If no pulmonary venous obstruction, asymptomatic at birth with eventual tachypnea, poor feeding, heart failure

      c. Murmurs absent with pulmonary venous obstruction, but grade II blowing systolic mumur heard best over xiphoid and left lower sternal border when no obstruction is present

      d. Electrocardiogram shows right atrial enlargement, severe right ventricular hypertrophy

      e. Chest film shows cardiomegaly with increased pulmonary vascularity

    4. Diagnosis

      a. Clinical symptoms and signs

      b. Chest film, electrocardiogram, echocardiogram

      c. Cardiac catheterization

    5. Complications

        Cardiac failure and death if not treated

    6. Treatment

        Atrial septostomy with subsequent surgical repair early in infancy

L. Tracheovascular Ring (Fig. 53)

    1. Definition and anatomy

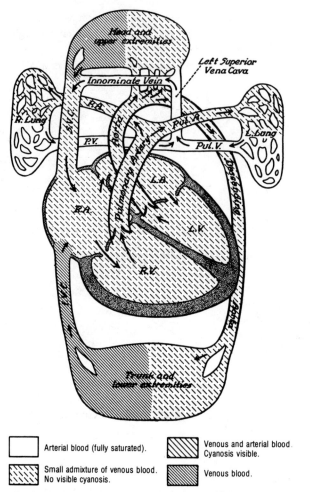

☐ Arterial blood (fully saturated).	▨ Venous and arterial blood. Cyanosis visible.
▧ Small admixture of venous blood. No visible cyanosis.	▩ Venous blood.

Fig. 52. Total anomalous pulmonary venous return. In this malformation, all the pulmonary veins drain into the right atrium instead of into the left atrium. In those instances in which only some of the pulmonary veins drain anomalously, the condition is termed *partial* rather than *total* anomalous pulmonary venous return. With *total* return, a number of routes of return may exist, but the hemodynamics are essentially the same. The anomalous connection may be to the right atrium, the right superior vena cava, the left innominate vein, the coronary sinus, or to the subdiaphragmatic channels (portal vein, ductus venosus, inferior vena cava, hepatic vein).

In this condition, blood can enter the left side of the heart only by way of an interatrial communication, so this is necessary for life. Because of volume overload of the right side of the heart, right atrial enlargement and right ventricular hypertrophy are present. Cyanosis is generally absent unless pulmonary venous obstruction is present. Pulmonary venous obstruction is commonly associated with the subdiaphragmatic anomalous connections and contributes to their poorer prognosis. (*Taussig HB: Congenital Malformations of the Heart, Vol. II, Specific Malformations, p 555. Cambridge, MA, Harvard Univ. Press, 1960*)

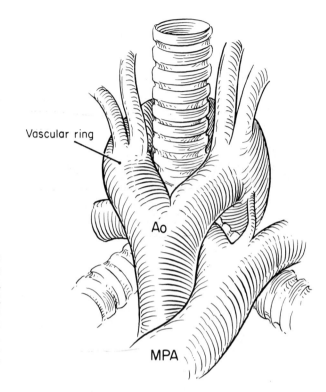

Fig. 53. Vascular ring due to double aortic arch. This abnormality results from failure of regression of the embryonic right eighth dorsal aortic segment. All reported cases have had a left-sided ductus arteriosus. The right and left aortic arches arise as branches of the ascending aorta, encircle the trachea and esophagus, and then unite posteriorly to form a single descending aorta. Cardiac hemodynamics remain normal, and there are no changes in the electrocardiogram or in cardiac function. Symptoms are related to mechanical compression of the trachea and not to altered cardiac physiology. **Ao,** aorta; **MPA,** main pulmonary artery. (*Moss AJ, McDonald LV: Cardiac disease in the wheezing child. Chest 71:187, 1977*)

  a. Vascular ring surrounding trachea and esophagus that may cause tracheal compression
  b. Due to abnormalities of aortic arch including double arched aorta and aberrant right subclavian artery
  2. Manifestations
  a. Wheezing, retractions, crowing stridor
  b. Recurrent pulmonary infections
  c. No murmurs
  d. Patients tend to lie with head and neck in hyperextended position
  3. Diagnosis
  a. Manifestations
  b. Barium-swallow roentgenogram
  c. Cardiac catheterization
  d. *Patient frequently diagnosed as having croup, bronchitis, or asthma*
  4. Treatment
     Surgery when diagnosis is established
M. Bicuspid Aortic Valve (Fig. 54)
  1. Definition
     Aortic valve has only two leaflets instead of customary three

A

Two cusps of equal
width and length

B

Two cusps equal in length
but unequal in width

C

Two cusps equal in
width but unequal
in length

D

Two cusps unequal
in both width and length

Fig. 54. Diagrammatic illustration of various types of bicuspid valves. All may be incompetent or stenotic, and all are prone to development of bacterial endocarditis. (*Moss AJ: What every primary physician should know about the postoperative cardiac patient.* Pediatrics 63:320, 1979; Copyright American Academy of Pediatrics 1979)

   2. Incidence and associated diseases
      a. Approximately 2% of general population
      b. Associated particularly with coarctation of aorta
   3. Manifestations
         Asymptomatic
   4. Diagnosis
      a. Echocardiography
      b. Cardiac catheterization (angiocardiography)
   5. Complications
      a. Aortic stenosis or aortic insufficiency
      b. Bacterial endocarditis
   6. Treatment
         None
 N. Mitral Valve Prolapse (Barlow's Syndrome, Floppy Mitral Valve)
   1. Definition and anatomy
      a. Disorder manifested by protrusion of posterior leaflet into left atrium durin
         systole
      b. Posterior leaflet demonstrates myxomatous degeneration
   2. Incidence and associated conditions
      a. Incidence increases with age
      b. Associated with atrial septal defect, osteogenesis imperfecta, Ehlers-Danlos
         syndrome, pseudoxanthoma elasticum, and Marfan's syndrome
      c. Probably the most common congenital cardiac lesion, occurring in about 5%
         of general population
   3. Manifestations
      a. May be completely asymptomatic
      b. Chest pain, fatigue, dyspnea

    c. Late systolic murmur and midsystolic click in mitral area

    d. Arrhythmias

  4. Diagnosis

    Phonocardiography, echocardiography, cardiac catheterization

  5. Complications (15%)

    a. Bacterial endocarditis

    b. Serious arrhythmia

    c. Marked mitral regurgitation

    d. Sudden death

  6. Treatment

    Antibiotic prophylaxis for those conditions that predispose to bacterial endocarditis

INNOCENT MURMURS

A. General Considerations

  1. Defined as murmurs not associated with any cardiac pathology and generally transient in nature

  2. Occur mainly in children 2–7 years

B. Vibratory Murmur

  1. Grade I–III, low pitched, early-to-mid-systolic murmur heard best over third and fourth left intercostal spaces

  2. Heard best with bell part of stethoscope

  3. Described as musical, fiddle-string, twanging-string in nature

  4. Lessens or even disappears when patient placed in upright position

C. Pulmonic Ejection Murmur

  1. Grade I–III, early-to-mid-systolic murmur heard best at second and third left intercostal spaces

  2. Thought to be caused by increased pulmonary flow (anxiety, anemia, or exercise)

  3. Must differentiate from atrial septal defect

    a. Widely split second sound on expiration and inspiration, abnormal electrocardiogram and chest film all favor atrial septal defect

    b. Normal electrocardiogram rules out *significant* atrial septal defect

D. Venous Hum

  1. Continuous, low-to-medium-pitched murmur, heard best at base of heart and over neck

  2. Sound louder if patient upright and louder in diastole

  3. Disappears when neck veins are occluded or patient turns head to side

E. Cardiorespiratory Murmur

  1. Occurs during mid-to-late systole, heard over any part of precordium

  2. Intensity varies with respiration

  3. Can be loud, high-pitched with almost screeching quality ("systolic whoop")

F. Carotid Bruits
1. Early-to-mid-systolic murmurs heard over right carotid artery (often associated with thrill)
2. Distinguished from aortic stenosis by absence over aortic area

ARRHYTHMIAS

A. Sinus Arrhythmia
1. Inspiration normally associated with faster heart rate than expiration. May result in irregular heart rate
2. More pronounced in children than adults
3. Of no clinical significance
4. Disappears with exercise
B. Sinus Tachycardia
Occurs in apprehension, exercise, fever, pain, crying, shock, anemia, infections, hyperthyroidism, myocarditis, with stimulants (alcohol, coffee, tobacco), drugs (epinephrine, atropine)
C. Sinus Bradycardia
Occurs in vagotonia, highly trained athletes, elevated intracranial pressure, sleep, myocarditis, hypothyroidism, drugs (digitalis, quinidine, anesthetic agents)
D. Extrasystoles
1. Are single or multiple premature contractions resulting from ectopic impulses in atria, atrioventricular node, or ventricles
2. May occur in normal hearts, particularly in adolescents
3. Precipitating factors include emotional stress, drugs, stimulants
4. Generally require no treatment
E. Paroxysmal Tachycardia
1. A series of ectopic beats occurring in rapid sequence
2. May be supraventricular (atrial or nodal) or ventricular in origin
3. Characterized by rapid regular heart rate
4. Diagnosis
Electrocardiogram
5. Must exclude associated heart disease
F. Atrial Flutter
1. Rapid regular atrial rhythm with atrial rate usually exceeding 300/min
2. Originates from atrial ectopic focus
3. Some degree of atrioventricular block commonly occurs, resulting in slower ventricular rate
4. Diagnosis
Electrocardiogram
5. Occurs in heart disease, cardiac tumors, digitalis intoxication, hyperthyroidism and in neonate with and without heart disease

G. Atrial Fibrillation
  1. Series of extremely rapid but irregular atrial contractions with totally irregular response of ventricles
  2. Atrial contractions originate from single focus or multiple foci in atria
  3. Atrial rate is 400–600/min with ventricular rate of 50–200/min
  4. Diagnosis
      Electrocardiogram
  5. Occurs with heart disease, cardiac tumors, digitalis intoxication, hyperthyroidism
  6. Must exclude associated heart disease

BLOOD PRESSURE MEASUREMENT

A. Errors in Measurement Relate to Patient, Instrument, Technique, or Examiner
B. Must Relieve Patient's Anxiety and Allow Time for Recovery from Recent Activity
C. Instrument Should Be Examined for Mechanical Defects
D. Mercury Level Should Be Vertical and Meniscus at Level of Examiner's Eye
E. Width of Cuff Should be Two-thirds Length of Upper Arm
F. Cuff Should Be Inflated Rapidly and Deflated Slowly (2–5 mm Hg per second)
G. Measurement by Ultrasound (Doppler technique) Is Reliable and Used in Intensive Care Units, Operating Rooms, and Neonatal Nursery

HEART FAILURE

A. Definition
  1. Represents inability of heart to meet metabolic requirements of body as manifested by clinical signs of pulmonary and systemic venous congestion
  2. Can arise from excessive workload caused by structural defect (*i.e.,* congenital aortic stenosis), intrinsic alterations of myocardium (*i.e.,* myocarditis), or from a combination
B. Manifestations
  1. Signs of impaired myocardial function
      Tachycardia, gallop rhythm, cold extremities, weak peripheral pulses, pulsus paradoxus, pulsus alternans,* cardiomegaly on roentgenogram
  2. Signs of pulmonary congestion
      Tachypnea, wheezes, rales, cyanosis, cough, dyspnea on exertion, paroxysmal nocturnal dyspnea
  3. Signs of systemic congestion
      a. Hepatomegaly most reliable sign
      b. Neck vein distention
      c. Peripheral edema (rare, poor prognosis)

* See Glossary

4. Electrocardiogram of little help
5. Echocardiography may assess myocardial function

C. Diagnosis

Clinical signs and symptoms

D. Treatment

1. Digitalis drug of choice
    a. *Digitalization*
        1. *Prematures:* 35 μg per kg IV or PO
        2. *Less than 2 years of age:* 50–70 μg per kg PO, IV 75% of PO dose
        3. *More than 2 years of age:* 30–50 μg per kg PO, IV 75% of PO dose (maximum total dose 1 mg)
    b. Maintenance dose ¼–⅓ of digitalization dose given in two divided doses/24 hours
    c. Monitor serum digitalis, electrolyte levels, electrocardiogram
2. Other inotropic drugs
    a. Isoproterenol or dopamine used in patients with severe heart failure with decreased peripheral perfusion
    b. Should be given by infusion pump with monitoring of central venous and wedge pressures
3. Diuretics
    a. Thiazides (hydrochlorthiazide)
        1. Promotes excretion of sodium, water, chloride, potassium
        2. Kaliuretic effect may be a problem
    b. Ethacrynic acid and furosemide (Lasix)
        1. More effective than thiazides
        2. Used extensively in acute heart failure
        3. Chronic use requires special attention to potassium loss
    c. Aldosterone antagonists (spironolactone)
        1. Cause sodium excretion and promote potassium retention
        2. Used in conjunction with thiazides, ethacrynic acid, or furosemide (tends to correct potassium loss)
        3. Important drug in chronic heart failure
    d. Complications of diuretic therapy
        1. *Dilutional hyponatremia:* Water retained more than salt. Treat by water restriction. Improvement of cardiac function returns electrolytes to normal balance
        2. *Hypokalemia:* Predisposes to digitalis toxicity. Administration of potassium supplement and/or spironolactone corrects problem
        3. *Hyperkalemia:* Occurs with spironolactone therapy or in patients who fail to respond to diuretic therapy
        4. *Acute sodium depletion:* Common problem. Symptoms include lethargy, drop in blood pressure, reduced skin turgor, edema
4. Oxygen
5. Bed rest
6. Steroids helpful in rheumatic carditis or viral myocarditis
7. Sedation with morphine sulfate reduces pulmonary edema
8. Treat underlying condition

BIBLIOGRAPHY

Isabel-Jones JB et al: Echocardiographic incidence of bicuspid aortic valve. Pediatr Dig 19:13–16, 1977

Malcolm AD et al: Clinical and investigative findings in presence of mitral leaflet prolapse. Study of 85 consecutive patients. Br Heart J 38:244–256, 1976

Moss AJ: Indirect methods of blood pressure measurement. Pediatr Clin North Am 25:3–14, 1978

Moss AJ: What every primary physician should know about the postoperative cardiac patient. Pediatrics 63:320–330, 1979

Moss AJ, Adams FH, Emmanouilides GC: Heart Disease in Infants, Children and Adolescents. Baltimore, Williams and Wilkins, 1977

Rudolph AM, Barnett HL, Einhorn AH: Pediatrics. New York, Appleton-Century-Crofts, 1977

7

Gastroenterology

CONGENITAL MALFORMATIONS

A. Tracheoesophageal Fistula (TEF, Fig. 55)
  1. Definition and anatomy
     a. Communication between esophagus and trachea. Is a result of incomplete separation of the embryonic foregut into esophagus and trachea at 4–6 weeks gestation
     b. Commonly associated with esophageal atresia, rarely seen alone
     c. Five recognized types of TEF and esophageal atresia
        1. TEF alone (4%)
        2. Esophageal atresia with distal TEF (most common form 86%)
        3. Esophageal atresia with proximal TEF (1%)
        4. Esophageal atresia with proximal and distal TEF (1%)
        5. Esophageal atresia alone (8%)
  2. Incidence and associations
     a. 1 of 2500–3000 births
     b. Polyhydramnios present in 85% of cases with esophageal atresia alone, 32% when TEF also present

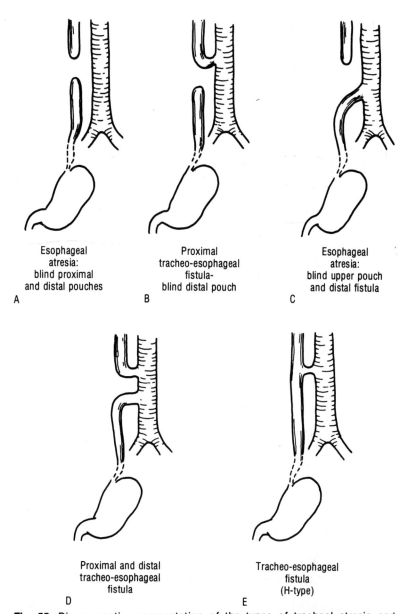

Esophageal
atresia:
blind proximal
and distal pouches

A

Proximal
tracheo-esophageal
fistula-
blind distal pouch

B

Esophageal
atresia:
blind upper pouch
and distal fistula

C

Proximal and distal
tracheo-esophageal
fistula

D

Tracheo-esophageal
fistula
(H-type)

E

Fig. 55. Diagrammatic representation of the types of tracheal atresia and tracheoesophageal fistulas. (*Gryboski J: Gastrointestinal Problems in the Infant, p 60. Philadelphia, W. B. Saunders, 1975*)

    c. Associated with anomalies of cardiovascular system, gastrointestinal tract (particularly imperforate anus), urinary tract

    d. Also associated with cleft lip and palate, Down's syndrome, trisomy 18

3. Manifestations

    a. 34% of infants are small for gestational age

    b. Excess salivation requiring frequent suctioning

    c. Choking, coughing, cyanosis in feeding

    d. Acute gastric distention

        Due to air entering stomach from fistula

    e. Pulmonary disease

        1. Atelectasis from mucus obstructing right upper lobe bronchus

        2. Pneumonia secondary to aspiration due to overflow from blind esophageal pouch or reflux through fistula from stomach (potentially lethal)

    f. Chest and abdominal films may show air-filled upper pouch

4. Diagnosis

    a. Clinical signs and symptoms

    b. Failure to pass cathether into stomach (esophageal atresia)

    c. Presence of air in stomach or intestines on roentgenogram establishes existence of lower TEF

    d. Contrast studies should be performed by experienced radiologist

        1. Lipid-containing contrast to be avoided because of risk of lipid pneumonitis

        2. Gastrografin not to be used because of hypertonicity (can cause large fluid shifts into bowel lumen)

        3. Small-particle-size barium is contrast of choice

5. Complications

    Aspiration pneumonia

6. Treatment

    a. Suction of upper pouch

    b. Immediate gastrostomy to decompress stomach

    c. Complete repair when patient's health permits

    d. Patient with pneumonitis requires proper supportive and antibiotic therapy before surgery

B. Bowel Obstruction

1. Definition

    Prevention of passage of food or meconium through bowel due to blockage or stenosis

2. Manifestations

    a. Maternal polyhydramnios

        1. Greater than 1500–2000 ml of amniotic fluid

        2. Occurs with high intestinal atresia

    b. Bilious vomiting

        Presence of bile in gastric aspirate or a volume of aspirate greater than 20 ml may signify obstruction

    c. Abdominal distention

      1. Severe distention may be associated with respiratory distress or with visible loops of bowel

      2. Gross distention usually associated with low obstruction

    d. Failure to pass meconium* in first 24 hours after birth (meconium ileus)

      1. Associated with low small-bowel obstruction, Hirschsprung's disease, colon atresia, meconium plug syndrome.*

      2. Also observed in nonobstructive diseases (*i.e.,* cystic fibrosis)

    e. Abdominal film may show dilated intestinal loops with air-fluid levels

  3. Diagnosis

    a. Clinical signs and symptoms

    b. Abdominal films and contrast studies

  4. Complications

      Perforation with subsequent peritonitis

  5. Treatment

    a. Decompression

      Nasogastric suction

    b. Surgical repair if necessary and if patient can tolerate procedure

C. Anorectal Anomalies

  1. Definition

    a. Structural abnormality of anus or rectum

    b. Five types recognized

      1. *Anal stenosis:* Small anal opening

      2. *Imperforate anus:* Membrane covering anus

      3. *Anal agenesis:* Small anal opening with intact external sphincter. Meconium and stool cannot pass (most common). Fistulas may be present

      4. *Anal and rectal agenesis:* Fistulas invariably present

      5. *Rectal atresia:* Anal canal and lower rectum form blind pouch

  2. Incidence and associations

    a. Occurs in 1 in 3000–4000 births

    b. Associated with TEF, sacral defects, atresias elsewhere in gastrointestinal tract (see Chap. 2)

  3. Manifestations

    a. Anal stenosis

      Passage of ribbonlike stool, fecal impaction, abdominal distention

    b. Other types of anorectal anomalies

      1. Failure to pass meconium, abdominal distention (if no fistulas present)

      2. If fistulas present may find meconium in urine or vagina

  4. Diagnosis

    a. Clinical signs and symptoms

    b. Roentgenogram with radiopaque object at normal anal opening can determine level of terminal bowel

    c. Ultrasound

* See Glossary

5. Complications
   Perforation with peritonitis
6. Treatment
   a. Nasogastric suction to decompress bowel if obstruction is present
   b. Stenotic anus may respond to digital dilatation
   c. Imperforate anus treated with excision of membrane and dilatation
   d. Colostomy treatment of choice for other types
   e. 20% mortality for anal and rectal agenesis

D. Diaphragmatic Hernia (Fig. 56)
   1. Definition and anatomy
      a. Protrusion of abdominal viscera into thoracic cavity through defect in diaphragm
      b. Most common type caused by incomplete closure of pleuroperitoneal sinus (foramen of Bochdalek, 80%)
         Foramen present bilaterally on posterolateral portion of diaphragm
      c. Can get herniation through substernal sinus (1%) or esophageal hiatus (15%)
      d. Hernias generally not surrounded by peritoneal sac (false hernia)
   2. Incidence and associations
      a. Present in 1 in 2200 births
      b. Left-sided hernia much more common
      c. Associated with malrotation, Meckel's diverticulum, patent ductus arteriosus, atrial septal defect (secundum type), coarctation of aorta, neurologic anomalies
   3. Manifestations
      a. Vary according to amount of abdominal viscera in thoracic cavity and type of defect
      b. Bochdalek hernia
         1. In high-risk cases, cyanosis, respiratory distress, poor feeding, tachypnea with substernal, intercostal retractions (develop within 72 hours after birth)
         2. Symptoms reduced in mild cases
         3. Physical findings include diminished or absent breath sounds on involved side, rales, flat abdomen, bowel sounds in thorax
      c. Hiatal hernia
         1. Vomiting from time of birth; may be projectile, occurs after feeding; vomitus can be blood-streaked; patient may develop torsion spasms of head and upper extremities (Sandifer's syndrome)*
         2. Physical findings same as Bochdalek hernia
      d. Substernal hernia
         1. Usually asymptomatic; vomiting may be present
         2. Discovered incidentally on chest film
      e. Chest film demonstrates bowel loops in thorax

* See Glossary

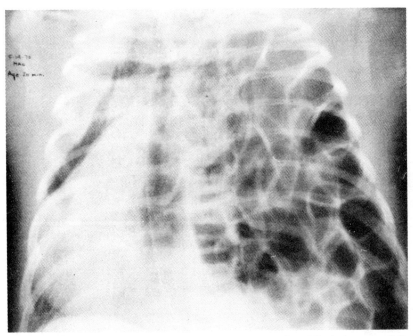

Fig. 56. Congenital diaphragmatic hernia in a newborn infant. The baby was mildly cyanotic at birth and became much worse when assisted ventilation was given through a face mask. The ventilatory assistance caused gaseous distention of the multiple small-bowel loops in the left chest with compromise of right lung function. A Bochdalek hernia was successfully repaired at surgery, but the patient subsequently died of persistent bronchopleural fistulas that developed in the hypoplastic left lung. (*Gryboski J: Gastrointestinal Problems in the Infant, p 74. Philadelphia, W. B. Saunders, 1975*)

4. Diagnosis
    a. Clinical signs and symptoms
    b. Chest film
5. Complications
    a. Hypoplastic lung
    b. Aspiration pneumonia
    c. Esophagitis with stricture
    d. Death (50% of high-risk infants)
6. Treatment
    a. Bochdalek and substernal hernia
        1. Nasogastric suction to decompress bowel
        2. Corrective surgery
    b. Hiatal hernia
        1. Place infant in upright position after feeding
        2. Corrective surgery if hematemesis, severe anemia, stricture formation

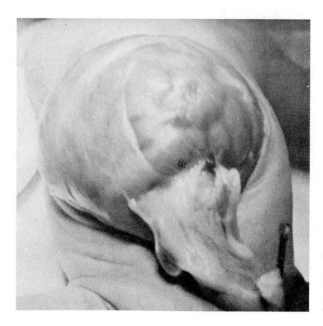

Fig. 57. Large omphalocele. Note the central insertion of cord. (Courtesy of L. Pickett, M.D.) (*Gryboski J: Gastrointestinal Problems in the Infant, p 215. Philadelphia, W. B. Saunders, 1975*)

E. Omphalocele (exomphalus, Fig. 57)
  1. Definition and anatomy
     a. Protrusion of intestine through large defect of abdominal wall into umbilical cord. Is due to early failure of rectus muscles to approach one another and close the circular defect after the midgut returns into the abdominal cavity from the umbilical cord
     b. External bowel covered only by *amnion and peritoneum*
  2. Incidence and associations
     a. Present in 1 of 3000–5000 births
     b. Associated with malrotation or bowel atresia (33%), cardiovascular anomalies, genitourinary anomalies, and Beckwith's syndrome*
  3. Manifestations
     a. Mostly premature infants
     b. Bowel visible on abdominal wall
  4. Diagnosis
     Clinical signs
  5. Complications
     a. Death (30% if small, 70% if large)
     b. Bowel infarction
     c. Peritonitis
     d. Intestinal obstruction

* See Glossary

6. Treatment
   a. Nasogastric suction to keep bowel decompressed
   b. Small defect can be closed primarily
   c. Large defect requires two-stage procedure (due to inadequate abdominal cavity)
      1. Large plastic sac constructed around omphalocele
      2. Omphalocele reduced over several days to weeks
      3. Abdominal wall defect closed after successful reduction

F. Gastroschisis (Fig. 58)
   1. Definition and anatomy
      a. Paraumbilical* defect in abdominal wall; usually associated with protrusion of bowel
      b. No sac covers bowel
      c. Most defects on right side
   2. Incidence and associations
      a. Present in 1 of 50,000 births
      b. Associated with malrotation and intestinal atresia (20%), prematurity (75%)
   3. Manifestations
      Edematous bowel protruding from abdomen
   4. Diagnosis
      Clinical signs
      Can be confused with ruptured omphalocele. Look for normal insertion of umbilical cord
   5. Complications
      a. Mortality 40%
      b. Bowel infarction
      c. Perforation with or without peritonitis
      d. Intestinal obstruction
   6. Treatment
      Same as for omphalocele

G. Absent Abdominal Musculature (Prune Belly, Fig. 59)
   1. Definition and anatomy
      a. Absence of lower rectus abdominis muscle and lower and medial oblique muscles with megaureters and bladder, hydronephrosis, cryptorchidism (see Chap. VIII). Failure to develop this musculature is probably the result of damage to the embryo during the second gestational month
      b. Variable degrees of syndrome
         1. Muscle mass may be present but hypoplastic
         2. Ureters and bladder may be only slightly dilated
   2. Incidence and associated conditions
      a. Rare
      b. Male preponderance
      c. Can be associated with dysplasia of kidneys, urethral atresia, or stenosis

* See Glossary

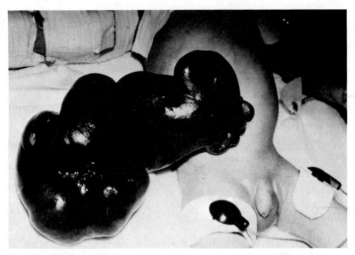

Fig. 58. Evisceration of the entire gastrointestinal tract of a newborn infant with gastroschisis. (*Avery GB (ed): Neonatology. Philadelphia, J. B. Lippincott, 1975*)

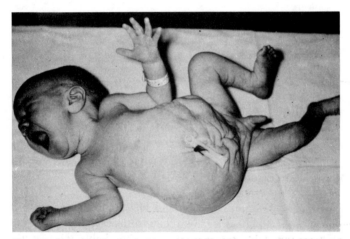

Fig. 59. Prune belly syndrome: typical appearance of the abdominal wall. (*Avery GB (ed): Neonatology. Philadelphia, J. B. Lippincott, 1975*)

3. Manifestations
   a. Large distended abdomen with wrinkling and creasing of skin
   b. History of multiple upper and lower respiratory infections, urinary tract infections
   c. Ineffective cough
   d. Palpable bladder and kidneys
   e. No resistance to abdominal palpation
   f. Abdominal film shows megalocystis and megaureters
4. Diagnosis
   a. Clinical signs and symptoms
   b. Abdominal film, pyelogram
5. Complications
   a. Urinary tract infections
   b. Hydronephrosis
   c. Renal failure
   d. Pneumonia
   e. Death (age depends on severity of disease)
6. Treatment
   a. Supportive for complications
   b. Girdle for abdomen
   c. Some surgeons advise urinary tract surgery to prevent reflux and reduce hydronephrosis

H. Errors in Rotation of Intestine
   1. Definition and anatomy
      a. Normally, intestine undergoes 270° counterclockwise rotation in the abdomen
      b. Nonrotation of midgut
         Midgut fails to rotate after reentering abdomen
      c. Incomplete duodenal rotation
         Duodenum does not rotate behind superior mesenteric artery
      d. Incomplete rotation of cecum
         1. Most common form of malrotation
         2. Cecum lies in right upper quadrant or midline
      e. Reversed rotation
         1. Midgut first rotates 90° *clockwise*, then 180° counterclockwise
         2. Cecum and transverse colon lie posterior to duodenum and superior mesenteric artery
   2. Incidence
      a. Unknown
      b. Approximately 2 : 1 male preponderance
   3. Manifestations
      a. Symptoms result from complications (duodenal obstruction, volvulus,* incarceration*)

* See Glossary

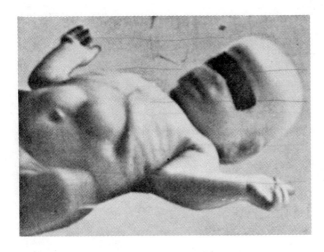

Fig. 60. Gastric peristaltic waves of pyloric stenosis in an infant 3 weeks of age. (*Courtesy of Dr. Carl Wagner, Cincinnati*) (*Barbero GJ: In Vaughan, VC III, McKay RJ, Nelson WE (eds): Nelson Textbook of Pediatrics, p 821. Philadelphia, W. B. Saunders, 1975*)

Bilious vomiting, abdominal distention, bloody stools (uncommon; associated with volvulus), jaundice
   b. Many infants symptomatic during first week of life
   c. Abdominal film shows dilated bowel with air fluid levels
  4. Diagnosis
    a. Clinical signs and symptoms
    b. Abdominal films
  5. Complications
    a. Intestinal obstruction
    b. Volvulus
    c. Incarceration of bowel
  6. Treatment
    a. Nasogastric suction
    b. Corrective surgery
 I. Hypertrophic Pyloric Stenosis
  1. Definition and anatomy
    Hypertrophied pyloric muscle causing stenosis of lumen and resulting in obstruction to passage of food
  2. Incidence
    a. About 1 per 500 births
    b. Approximately 4 : 1 male to female ratio
    c. Familial disorder
       Increased incidence if one parent had disease
  3. Manifestations
    a. Symptoms usually begin at 2–6 weeks
    b. Projectile vomiting, weight loss, ravenous appetite
    c. Visible abdominal peristaltic waves (Fig. 60)
    d. Abdominal mass (size of olive) may be palpated

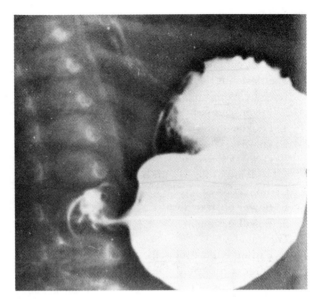

Fig. 61. Hypertrophic pyloric stenosis. Note the elongated, narrow pyloric canal (string sign) as well as the blunt antrum. The base of the duodenal bulb is concave. Hyperperistalsis was noted fluoroscopically. (*Barbero GJ: In Vaughan VC III, McKay RJ, Nelson WE (eds): Nelson Textbook of Pediatrics, p 822. Philadelphia, W. B. Saunders, 1975*)

     e. Barium-contrast roentgenogram shows dilated stomach with narrow pylorus ("string sign," Fig. 61)

4. Diagnosis
   a. Clinical signs and symptoms
   b. Typical "olive" mass
   c. X-ray examination
5. Complications
   a. Dehydration
   b. Metabolic alkalosis ✓   *loss of H^+*   *HypoCl*
   c. Electrolyte imbalance
6. Treatment
   a. Nasogastric suction
   b. Correct alkalosis and electrolyte imbalance
   c. Pyloromyotomy (Ramstedt operation)

INTUSSUSCEPTION

A. Definition and Anatomy
1. Invagination (telescoping) of one part of intestine into lumen of adjacent part
2. Generally originates in ileum
3. Lead points include Meckel's diverticula, polyps, intraluminal cysts, foci of lymphoid hyperplasia

B. Incidence
 1. About twice as common in boys
 2. Rare in first month of life
 3. Most commonly occurs between 1 month and 2 years of age
C. Manifestations
 1. Colic, vomiting, grossly bloody stools ("currant jelly stools")   ✓✓
 2. Fever, tachycardia, mass in right lower abdominal quadrant   *intermittent pain*
 3. Leukocytosis
D. Diagnosis
 1. Clinical signs and symptoms
 2. Abdominal films with barium enema
E. Complications
 1. Bowel obstruction
 2. Bowel gangrene
F. Treatment
 1. Barium enema reduces intussusception in many instances
 2. Surgery indicated when barium-enema reduction is unsuccessful, toxic clinical state, signs of peritonitis, or evidence of intestinal obstruction

MECKEL'S DIVERTICULUM

A. Definition and Anatomy
 1. Remnant of omphalomesenteric duct (vitelline duct)
 2. Ectopic gastric, duodenal, or pancreatic tissue may be present
B. Incidence
  "Rule of two"—In 2% of population, twice as common in males, peak incidence at 2 years of age
C. Manifestations
  Three types of presentations
  a. Hemorrhage
    Can be massive (usually painless) rectal bleeding. May develop shock. Gastric mucosa with ulcer on opposite ileal mucosa usually present
  b. Intestinal obstruction
    1. *Intussusception:* May act as lead point causing intussusception and obstruction
    2. *Volvulus:* Fibrous band connecting diverticulum to abdominal wall may strangulate bowel causing pain, abdominal distention, bloody stools
  c. Diverticulitis
    Fever, vomiting, right lower quadrant pain, leukocytosis (simulates appendicitis). Rigid abdomen if perforation occurs
D. Diagnosis
 1. Clinical signs and symptoms
 2. Radionuclide scan of abdomen (technetium) to demonstrate ectopic gastric mucosa   *Meckel's scan*

E. Complications
  1. Perforation with peritonitis
  2. Bowel strangulation
  3. Hemorrhage
  4. Intussusception
  5. Volvulus
  6. Death
F. Treatment
  Surgery

HIRSCHSPRUNG'S DISEASE
(CONGENITAL AGANGLIONIC MEGACOLON)

Parasymph

A. Definition and anatomy
  1. Absence of parasympathetic ganglion cells in distal colon causing dilatation
  2. Involved area usually limited to bowel distal to sigmoid colon
B. Incidence
  Occurs in 1 in 5000 births
C. Manifestations
  1. Failure to pass meconium, vomiting, abdominal distention
  2. Symptoms may appear later and be related to partial obstruction
     Infrequent loose stolls with bilious vomiting, constipation
  3. May develop episodes of enterocolitis (fever, liquid diarrhea with severe dehydration)
  4. Stools ribbonlike, abdomen enlarged, palpable fecal masses
  5. Digital examination reveals no stool in anal canal
  6. Abdominal film shows dilated colon with narrowed distal segment (Fig. 62)
D. Diagnosis
  1. Clinical signs and symptoms
  2. Rectal biopsy
E. Complications
  Intestinal obstruction
F. Treatment
  Surgery

GASTROESOPHAGEAL REFLUX (G-E REFLUX)

A. Definition and Anatomy
  1. Retrograde flow of gastric contents into esophagus
  2. Due to incompetent lower esophageal sphincter
  3. Commonly associated with hiatal hernia

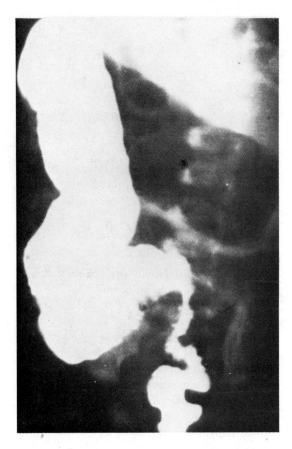

Fig. 62. Barium enema demonstrating the typical narrow distal rectal segment and proximal dilatation of Hirschsprung's disease. (*Martin LW: In Shirkey HC (ed): Pediatric Therapy, p 1086. Saint Louis, C. V. Mosby, 1975*)

B. Manifestations
  1. Vomiting, dysphagia, hematemesis, substernal pain, failure to thrive
  2. Malnutrition (below 15th percentile of height and weight)
  3. Anemia
C. Diagnosis
  1. Clinical signs and symptoms
  2. Barium-swallow studies
  3. Esophageal manometry
  4. Tuttle test*
D. Complications
  1. Esophagitis
  2. Esophageal stricture
  3. Bronchitis or asthma
  4. Toricollis (Sandifer's syndrome*)

  * See Glossary

E. Treatment
  1. Medical management
     a. Upright position after meals
     b. Antacids
  2. Surgery if medical management fails

PEPTIC ULCER DISEASE

A. Definition
   Erosion of mucous membrane of esophagus, stomach, or duodenum caused by
   gastric secretions
B. Incidence
  1. In infants, ulcer usually gastric
  2. In later life, duodenal ulcer more common

C. Manifestations
  1. Young infant
     a. Hematemesis, melena, perforation, shock
     b. May present as high intestinal obstruction (rare)
  2. Older infant and child
     Epigastric pain that may or may not be relieved by eating
D. Diagnosis
  1. Clinical signs and symptoms
  2. Upper gastrointestinal barium study
  3. Endoscopy
E. Complications
  1. Hemorrhage
  2. Perforation
  3. Obstruction
  4. Death
F. Treatment
  1. Antacid therapy
  2. Cimetidine
  3. Perforation requires immediate surgery
  4. Hemorrhage requires transfusions and surgery if bleeding cannot be controlled

ULCERATIVE COLITIS

A. Definition
   Chronic inflammation of colonic mucous membranes marked by chronicity with
   acute exacerbations
B. Pathology
  1. Rectum and distal colon usually involved but can extend into small intestine
  2. Inflammation usually limited to mucosa but can involve entire wall

C. Manifestations
1. Diarrhea, abdominal pain, rectal bleeding
2. Anorexia, weight loss, nausea, vomiting, malaise may also be present
3. Moderate abdominal tenderness on palpation
4. Extraintestinal manifestations include erythema multiforme,* erythema nodosum,* pyoderma gangrenosum*
5. Barium enema may be normal early in disease. Later, shaggy, barium-filled ulcerations are seen
6. Sigmoidoscopy shows hyperemic friable mucosa that bleeds easily

D. Diagnosis
1. Clinical signs and symptoms
2. Barium enema
3. Sigmoidoscopy

E. Complications
1. Arthritis
2. Liver disease
3. Iritis
4. Carcinoma of involved bowel

F. Treatment
1. Hospitalization for initial evaluation or if clinically toxic
2. Corticosteroid therapy only if disease is severe
3. Azulfidine may be helpful
4. Unrestricted diet
5. Supplemental vitamins if malnourished
6. Surgery if:
   a. Unresponsive to medical therapy
   b. Perforation
   c. Growth failure lasting 2–4 years
7. Psychotherapy for adjustment to chronic illness

CROHN'S DISEASE (REGIONAL ENTERITIS, GRANULOMATOUS COLITIS)

A. Definition
Chronic inflammatory disease of bowel
B. Pathology
1. Ileum most frequently involved
2. Disease may affect colon alone or in association with ileal disease
3. Areas of normal mucosa ("skip areas") between diseased segments
4. Involvement usually transmural
5. Histologic examination reveals multiple granulomas

* See Glossary

C. Manifestations
   1. Begins in preadolescence
   2. Onset can be sudden and mimic appendicitis
   3. Onset usually gradual
   4. Fever with or without abdominal pain
   5. Diarrhea, intermittent constipation, anorexia, periumbilical pain
   6. Anal fissures, fistulas, intestinal obstruction
   7. Growth failure
   8. Barium enema shows ulcerations, fistulas, pseudodiverticulitis
D. Diagnosis
   1. Clinical signs and symptoms
   2. Barium enema
   3. Sigmoidoscopy
E. Complications
   1. Hemorrhage
   2. Perforation
F. Treatment
   1. Corticosteroids for serious disease
   2. No good treatment available
   3. Surgery for fistulas, intestinal obstruction

APPENDICITIS

A. Definition
   Inflammation of appendix
B. Pathogenesis
   1. Obstruction is primary event that leads to appendicitis
   2. Obstruction may be secondary to inflammatory changes, fecalith,* pinworms, foreign body, stenosis, or kinking
C. Manifestations
   1. Periumbilical pain shifting to right lower quadrant with nausea, vomiting, anorexia, and low-grade fever is classic pattern
      Seen most often in older children
   2. Symptoms depend on position of appendix
   3. Majority of children under 5 years of age often have perforation and peritonitis when first seen (rigid abdomen, grunting respirations, fever, diarrhea)
   4. Leukocytosis
   5. Abdominal film may demonstrate fecalith
D. Diagnosis
   1. Clinical signs and symptoms
   2. Abdominal film

* See Glossary

E. Complications
   1. Perforation
   2. Peritonitis
   3. Thrombophlebitis (uncommon)
F. Treatment
   1. Peritonitis requires immediate preoperative antibiotic therapy
   2. Appendectomy treatment of choice

ANAL FISSURES

A. Definition
   Linear tear at mucocutaneous rim of anus
B. Pathogenesis
   Usually caused by passage of large, hard stools but can be due to anal stenosis or
   trauma
C. Clinical Manifestations
   1. Pain on defecation
   2. Withholding of stools
   3. Bright red blood after bowel movement
   4. Fissure usually visible on inspection
D. Diagnosis
   Manifestations
E. Complications
   Persistence of fissures
F. Treatment
   1. Stool softeners (most fissures heal with relief of constipation)
   2. Surgery for chronic cases

DIARRHEA

A. Milk Allergy
   1. Definition
      Hypersensitivity to cow's milk protein
   2. Incidence
      a. Frequently overdiagnosed
      b. Usually in early infancy
   3. Manifestations
      Diarrhea (may include blood and mucus), vomiting, abdominal pain, asso-
      ciated allergic disease (allergic rhinitis, bronchial asthma, atopic dermatitis,
      urticaria, anaphylaxis)
   4. Diagnosis
      a. Clinical signs and symptoms
      b. Challenge to cow's milk protein

5. Complications

Acquired lactase deficiency, gluten sensitivity, other disaccharidase deficiency (temporary)

6. Treatment

Eliminate milk from diet

B. Milk-Associated Gastroenteropathy

1. Definition

Protein-losing enteropathy in young children or infants after ingestion of milk

2. Manifestations

a. Watery diarrhea (may be bloody), heavy protein loss

b. Patient may be edematous, anemic

3. Diagnosis

Clinical signs and symptoms

4. Complications

a. Anemia

b. Hypoalbuminemia

5. Treatment

Elimination of milk products from diet

C. Disaccharidase Deficiencies

1. Definition

a. Absent or reduced quantity of intestinal disaccharidase

b. Lactase deficiency most common

c. Four main types of lactase deficiency

1. *Developmental:* Seen in premature and small-for-date infants

2. *Congenital:* Rare

3. *Late onset:* Hereditary, presents at about 5 years of age

4. *Secondary:* Due to injury to small-intestinal mucosa (milk allergy or infection)

2. Manifestations

Symptoms variable

1. Watery explosive diarrhea, abdominal distention, vomiting, failure to thrive or

2. Intermittent diarrhea, normal growth and weight

3. Diagnosis

a. Clinical signs and symptoms

b. Lactose tolerance test

Measurement of blood glucose at given intervals following lactose ingestion*

4. Treatment

a. Developmental, secondary types

1. Temporary removal of lactose from diet

* Positive test if blood glucose level does not rise more than 20 mg/dl, reducing substance in stool exceeds 0.25% and *pH* of stool is less than 6

        2. Resume lactose 4–8 weeks after cessation of illness
    b. Congenital and late onset types
        Permanent elimination of lactose from diet
D. Celiac Sprue
    1. Definition
        a. Enteropathy caused by gluten (in wheat) ingestion. Confined to proximal small bowel and usually induces malabsorption, biochemical, and clinical abnormalities
        b. Elimination of dietary gluten causes complete remission
        c. Gluten sensitivity persists throughout life
        d. Symptoms may present anytime during life
    2. Pathology
        Villous atrophy of proximal small-bowel mucosa
    3. Manifestations
        a. Majority of children present prior to 2 years of age
        b. Abnormal stools, anorexia, muscle wasting, vomiting, abdominal distention
        c. May present with irritability, apathy, hypotonia, retarded motor development
    4. Diagnosis
        a. Clinical signs and symptoms
        b. Small-bowel biopsy
        c. Therapeutic trial
    5. Complications
        a. Rickets, osteoporosis
        b. Hypoproteinemia
        c. Anemia
        d. Milk intolerance
        e. Lymphoma, carcinoma
    6. Treatment
        Gluten-free diet

FOREIGN BODIES

A. General Considerations
    1. Foreign bodies often pass through gastrointestinal tract uneventfully
    2. Long sharp objects are dangerous and require removal by endoscopy
    3. For dangerous foreign body that has passed stomach
        a. Follow object's progress with serial roentgenograms
        b. Examine every stool for foreign body
B. Bezoars
    1. Tumor mass in stomach comprised of hair (trichobezoar) or food (phytobezoar)
    2. In infants, children (especially mentally retarded or emotionally disturbed)
    3. Manifestations include gastric distress, indigestion, moveable abdominal mass, loss of hair (if patient pulls out and swallows hair)

4. Diagnosis by clinical signs and symptoms, upper gastrointestinal barium roentgenograms
5. Part of bezoar may dislodge and cause obstruction in lower intestine
6. Surgery required

PANCREATITIS

A. General Considerations
  1. Definition
     Inflammation of pancreas
  2. Incidence
     a. Occurs in all age groups
     b. Less frequent in pediatric population
  3. Manifestations
     a. Upper abdominal pain, fever, vomiting
     b. Physical findings vary from mild distress and irritability to shock, rebound tenderness, ileus, excessive guarding
     c. Ecchymosis of flank (Grey Turner's sign) or the umbilicus (Cullen's sign) uncommon
     d. Leukocytosis, elevated serum amylase, hyperbilirubinemia, hyperglycemia, hypocalcemia

  4. Diagnosis
     a. Clinical signs and symptoms
     b. Serum and urine amylase (amylase clearance test)
     c. Ultrasonography
     d. Abdominal film
  5. Complications
     a. Acute pancreatitis
        1. Shock
        2. Pseudocyst due to leakage of pancreatic fluid
        3. Abscess
        4. Hemorrhagic pancreatitis
     b. Chronic pancreatitis
        1. Diabetes mellitus
        2. Pseudocyst
        3. Intestinal malabsorption
  6. Treatment
     a. Acute form responds to medical management and is self-limited
     b. Hospitalization
     c. Analgesics
        1. Meperidine (Demerol)   MS causes sphincter of Oddi spw
        2. Morphine contraindicated because induces spasms of ampulla of Vater and may aggravate disease

       d. Fluid therapy

       e. Nasogastric suction

B. Drug-Induced Pancreatitis

    Steroids and cytotoxic drugs most common

C. Traumatic Pancreatitis

    1. Pancreatic injury occurs in small percentage of all abdominal trauma

    2. Bicycle injuries (handle bars) frequently implicated

    3. Symptoms may evolve slowly

    4. Pseudocyst complicates approximately one-third of cases

    5. May require subtotal pancreatectomy

D. Obstructive Pancreatitis

    1. Due to obstruction of pancreatic duct

    2. Causes include choledochal cyst, stenosis of ampulla of Vater, ascariasis, pseudocyst

    3. Treatment generally surgical

E. Pancreatitis Related to Infection

    1. Occurs with some viral diseases

       a. Mumps most frequently implicated

       b. Can occur with rubeola, rubella, coxsackie B, hepatitis B viruses

    2. Symptoms usually appear about 5 days after onset of illness

    3. Complications include hemorrhage, diabetes mellitus

F. Cystic Fibrosis

    1. May be associated with recurrent attacks of acute pancreatitis

    2. Etiology unknown

    3. Attacks usually preceded by fatty food, alcohol, or tetracycline ingestion

G. Familial Hereditary Pancreatitis

    1. Autosomal dominant, incomplete penetrance

    2. Recurrent episodes of nausea, vomiting, and epigastric pain

    3. Attacks may occur 1–2 times a month

    4. Diagnosis frequently not made until adult life

    5. Abdominal film demonstrates pancreatic calcifications

    6. Complications include diabetes mellitus (less frequently seen in alcoholic pancreatitis), pseudocysts, portal vein or splenic vein thrombosis

    7. Associated with increased incidence of malignant pancreatic tumors

H. Hemorrhagic Pancreatitis

    1. Serious form of pancreatitis

    2. Patient usually presents with severe symptoms, shock may dominate

    3. Prognosis grave

    4. Complications include ascites, vascular collapse, renal failure

I. Pancreatic Pseudocyst

    1. Secondary to pancreatic secretions escaping into lesser sac of omentum

    2. Vary in size from small to large

    3. Contain plasma, blood, pancreatic fluid, inflammatory debris

    4. Presumably caused by obstruction of pancreatic duct

5. Abdominal trauma most frequent cause
6. Abdominal mass and distention accompany symptoms of pancreatitis
7. Complications include infection, abscess, perforation, massive hemorrhage, bile duct obstruction, intestinal obstruction
8. Treatment
   a. Small pseudocyst treated medically
   b. Large pseudocyst should be surgically drained or excised (subtotal pancreatectomy)

HERNIAS (ABDOMINAL)

A. Definition
   Projection of abdominal contents through defect in peritoneal wall
B. Umbilical Hernia
   1. Definition
      a. Protrusion of abdominal contents into umbilicus due to incomplete fascial closure of umbilical ring
      b. Hernia entirely covered by skin and subcutaneous tissue
   2. Incidence and associated conditions
      a. Premature infants have high incidence (about 20–85%, depending on birth weight)
      b. More common in blacks and females
      c. Associated with Down's syndrome, Hurler's syndrome, hypothyroidism
   3. Manifestations
      a. Visible at birth
      b. Usually asymptomatic
      c. Can cause symptoms if bowel obstruction or strangulation* occurs (extremely rare)
   4. Diagnosis
      Clinical signs
   5. Complications (extremely rare)
      a. Obstruction
      b. Strangulation
   6. Treatment
      a. Vast majority close spontaneously
      b. Surgery indicated if bowel obstruction or strangulation occurs
      c. Surgery may be needed if defect persists after 4 years of age
C. Inguinal Hernia
   1. Definition
      a. *Direct:* Projection of abdominal contents through defect in inguinal canal
      b. *Indirect:* Peritoneal contents leave abdomen at deep inguinal ring
         Most common type in pediatric patients

* See Glossary

2. Incidence
   a. Incidence less than 1%
   b. More common in boys
   c. May occur at any age but most commonly during first few months of life
3. Manifestations
   a. Soft lump in groin
   b. Usually asymptomatic
   c. Can develop vomiting and abdominal distention if incarceration occurs
4. Diagnosis
   Manifestations
5. Complications
   a. Incarceration
   b. Obstruction
   c. Strangulation
6. Treatment
   a. Elective surgery for uncomplicated hernia
      1. Some surgeons prefer exploration of both sides because of high incidence of bilaterality
      2. Inguinal mass in females may represent prolapsed ovary but testis (testicular feminization syndrome*) may be found at operation
   b. Incarcerated hernia
      1. Sedation, Trendelenburg position,* manual reduction
      2. If reduction unsuccessful or if strangulation suspected, immediate surgery indicated
D. Femoral Hernia
   1. Definition
      Protrusion of abdominal contents into femoral canal
   2. Extremely rare in pediatric patients

CONSTIPATION

A. Definition
   Hard stools, difficult to pass, usually infrequent
B. Manifestations
   1. Infrequent hard stools, painful defecation, blood-streaked stools if anal fissures present
   2. Fecal impaction
C. Diagnosis
   1. Signs and symptoms
   2. May be confused with Hirschsprung's disease
D. Treatment
   1. Infants

* See Glossary

a. Prunes, prune juice, fruits
b. Stool softeners
2. Older children
a. Bowel Training (attempt to deficate should be made after breakfast every morning)
b. Mineral oil
c. In selected cases, psychiatric counseling may be required
d. *Continued use of enemas or laxatives should be discouraged*

BIBLIOGRAPHY

Evans HE, Glass L: Perinatal Medicine. Hagerstown, Harper and Row, 1976

Franken EA JR: Gastrointestinal Radiology in Pediatrics. Hagerstown, Harper & Row, 1975

Gryboski J: Gastrointestinal Problems in the Infant. Philadelphia, W. B. Saunders, 1975

Hockelman RA: Principles of Pediatrics. Health Care of the Young. New York, McGraw-Hill, 1978

Lebenthal E: Digestive Diseases in Children. New York, Grune & Stratton, 1978

Redo SF: Atlas of Surgery in the First Six Months of Life. Hagerstown, Harper & Row, 1978

Rudolph AM, Barnett HL, Einhorn WE: Pediatrics. New York, Appleton-Century-Crofts, 1977

Vaughan VC III, McKay RJ, Nelson WE: Nelson Textbook of Pediatrics. Philadelphia, W. B. Saunders, 1975

Disorders of the Genitourinary System

CONGENITAL MALFORMATIONS

A. Polycystic Disease
   1. Usually fatal hereditary renal disease in which both kidneys are studded with cysts (gross and microscopic)
   2. Death due to renal failure
   3. Death may occur early in life or patient may survive into adult life
B. Oculocerebrorenal Syndrome (Lowe's Syndrome)
   1. An X-linked recessive disorder with anomalies of eyes, brain, kidneys
   2. Degree of mental retardation and physical manifestations variable
   3. Hypotonia common finding
C. Horseshoe Kidney (Fused Kidneys, Fig. 63)
   1. Occurs in 1 in 600 births. Results from fusion of ureteric buds during embryonic life
   2. Kidneys fused and fail to ascend
   3. Many function normally and require no treatment
   4. Ureteral duplication with obstruction commonly present and requires surgical correction

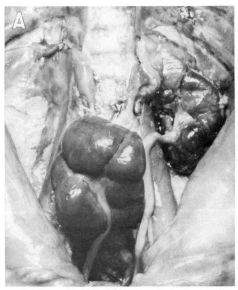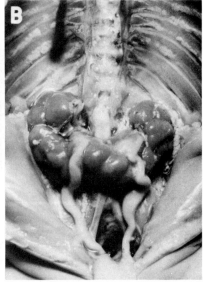

Fig. 63. (A) Displacement of right kidney with anterior rotation of the pelvis. **(B)** Horseshoe kidney *in situ* showing typical fusion of the lower poles with ureters crossing the anterior surfaces to reach the bladder. (*Reproduced with permission from Potter EL, Craig JM: Pathology of the Fetus and the Infant, 3rd edition. Copyright © 1975 by Year Book Medical Publishers, Inc., Chicago*)

D. Ectopic Kidney
    1. Usual site is pelvis. Kidney retains its low position of embryonic life
    2. Contralateral kidney usually normally placed
    3. Commonly associated with vesicoureteral reflux, ureteropelvic or ureteral obstruction
    4. May be associated with anorectal anomalies
E. Hydronephrosis (Fig. 64)
    1. Encountered at all ages but most commonly during first 6 months
    2. Definition
        Distention of renal pelvis and calyces with resultant pressure atrophy of renal parenchyma
    3. Results from obstruction of urinary tract (ureteropelvic junction, ureters, ureterovesical junction, urethra)
    4. Manifestations
        a. Flank mass (is most common abdominal mass in newborn)
        b. May have flank pain, hematuria, intercurrent urinary tract infections
    5. Diagnosis
        a. Established by intravenous urography
        b. Vesicoureteral reflux may be seen on retrograde cystourethrogram, depending on site of obstruction

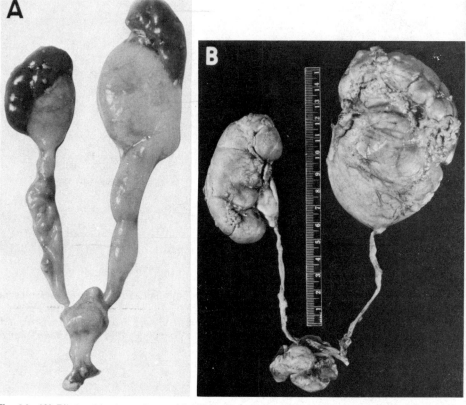

Fig. 64. (A) Bilateral hydroureter and hydronephrosis associated with moderate stenosis at the ureterovesical orifices. Stillborn fetus. **(B)** Massive dilatation of the pelvis of one kidney associated with local stenosis of the ureter. Infant aged 2 days. (*Reproduced with permission from Potter EL, Craig JM: Pathology of the Fetus and the Infant, 3rd edition. Copyright © 1975 by Year Book Medical Publishers, Inc., Chicago*)

      6. Treatment
        a. Surgical relief of obstruction
        b. Nephrectomy may be required
  F. Ureteral Duplication (Fig. 65)
      1. Many duplicated ureters function normally, but poor peristalsis above site of bifurcation and vesicoureteral reflux with intercurrent urinary tract infection not uncommon. This anomaly is produced by multiple ureteral buds originating from the mesonephric duct. *Incomplete* duplication results from early division of developing ureter and is *usually* asymptomatic
      2. Intravenous or retrograde urography establishes diagnosis
  G. Epispadias (Fig. 66)
      1. Urethra opens on dorsum of penis—confined to glans or may extend proximally. Is due to failure or incomplete closure of urogenital groove distally

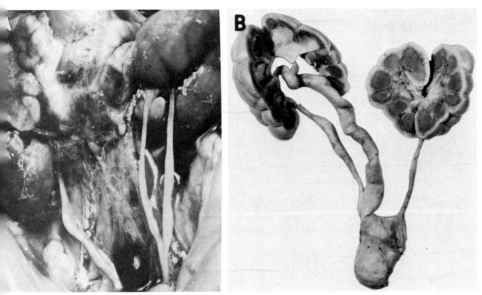

Fig. 65. Double ureter. **(A)** Unilateral branching of one ureter a short distance from the bladder. The kidney is more spherical than normal, and the pelvis is rotated anteriorly. **(B)** Unilateral double ureter with each orifice of the double ureter opening into separate kidney pelves. The ureter emptying into the upper pelvis is moderately dilated. (*Reproduced with permission from Potter EL, Craig JM: Pathology of the Fetus and the Infant, 3rd edition. Copyright © 1975 by Year Book Medical Publishers, Inc., Chicago*)

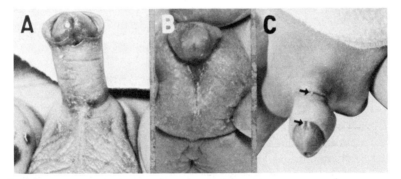

Fig. 66. Abnormal location of urethral meatus. **(A)** Mild hypospadias with slight downward displacement of urethral meatus. **(B)** Complete hypospadias with urethral meatus at the base of an abnormally short penis. **(C)** Epispadias with two accessory urethral orifices on the dorsum of the penis, one at the junction of the glans and prepuce and one in the area visible as a fold of skin near the base of the penis. (*Reproduced with permission from Potter EL, Craig JM: Pathology of the Fetus and the Infant, 3rd edition. Copyright © 1975 by Year Book Medical Publishers, Inc., Chicago*)

2. May be associated with chordee*
3. May be corrected surgically
H. Hypospadias (Fig. 66)
  1. Urethra opens on ventral side of penis. Is due to failure or incomplete closure of urogenital groove distally
  2. Most are minor glandular or subcoronal types
  3. May be associated with chordee, cryptorchidism, meatal stenosis
  4. Chordee requires surgical straightening of penis
  5. May be corrected surgically
I. Extrophy of Bladder (Ectropion, Fig. 67)
  1. Bladder is small with anterior surface exposed on abdominal wall. Is due to incomplete midline closure of lower part of abdominal wall in embryonic life. Involves abdominal wall, bladder, urethra, penis or clitoris, labia
  2. Associated with urinary incontinence, ulceration of bladder mucosa
  3. Results of reconstructive surgery usually unsatisfactory
J. Posterior Urethral Valves
  1. Causes obstruction of posterior urethra, often with ureteral reflux, hydro-ureters, and hydronephrosis
  2. Failure to thrive, renal failure, overflow dribbling, recurrent urinary infections usually appear during first year of life
  3. Treatment is surgical
K. Phimosis
  1. Definition
      Small preputial opening so that prepuce cannot be retracted over glans penis
  2. Treatment by forceful retraction usually sufficient
  3. If prepuce is retracted and cannot be replaced, then *paraphimosis* results. Latter characterized by edema, cyanosis, and even gangrene of glans penis. If prepuce cannot be replaced, incision of prepuce is required with circumcision after inflammation subsides

ACUTE GLOMERULONEPHRITIS

A. Clinical and Laboratory Features
  1. Oliguria*
  2. Edema
  3. Hypertension
  4. Hematuria and granular casts
  5. Proteinuria
  6. Azotemia
  7. Anemia
  8. Electrolyte and acid–base disturbances
  9. Increased erythrocyte sedimentation rate

* See Glossary

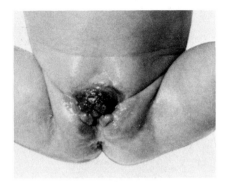

Fig. 67. Ectropion of the bladder. Female with separation of the two halves of the clitoris. (*Reproduced with permission from Potter EL, Craig JM: Pathology of the Fetus and the Infant, 3rd edition. Copyright © 1975 by Year Book Medical Publishers, Inc., Chicago*)

B. Poststreptococcal Glomerulonephritis
  1. Results from preceding pharyngeal or cutaneous infection with nephritogenic strains of group A beta-hemolytic streptococci [usually types 1, 3, 4, 12 with pharyngeal infection and 2, 49, 55, 57 with cutaneous infection (impetigo)]
  2. Manifestations
    a. As previously described for acute glomerulonephritis
    b. C_3 complement reduced
    c. Urine usually tea-colored with red cells, white cells, casts
  3. Diagnosis
    a. Clinical and laboratory manifestations
    b. History of preceding streptococcal infection with latent period
    c. May have high titer of antistreptococcal antibodies (ASO, antihyaluronidase, anti-DPNase)
    d. Renal biopsy only rarely indicated
  4. Course
    Most children return to usual state of health within 3–4 weeks, but microscopic urinary abnormalities may persist for 2 months or more
  5. Treatment
    a. Hospitalization required for renal failure, fluid and electrolyte disturbances, hypertension, hypertensive encephalopathy, pulmonary edema
    b. If general condition satisfactory, hospitalization not indicated and bed rest need not be enforced

CHRONIC GLOMERULONEPHRITIS

A. General Considerations
  1. Includes a variety of nonspecific diseases with progressive destruction of renal nephrons and ultimate renal insufficiency
  2. Also may be associated with systemic diseases such as anaphylactoid purpura (Henoch-Schönlein disease), diabetes mellitus, lupus erythematosis (see Chaps. IX, XI, XVII)

3. Is a feature of Alport's Syndrome (impaired hearing and chronic glomerulo-nephritis)
B. Laboratory Features
   1. Protineuria most common finding
   2. Microscopic red blood cells and leukocytes in urine
   3. Progressive deterioration of renal function
C. Diagnosis
   Renal biopsy extremely helpful
D. Prognosis
   1. Course is variable
   2. Azotemia is ominous sign, but survival for many years occasionally occurs
E. Treatment
   1. Symptomatic
   2. Dialysis or renal transplant in selected cases

IDIOPATHIC NEPHROTIC SYNDROME

A. General Considerations
   1. Characterized by proteinuria, hypoproteinemia, hyperlipemia, and edema. Recognizable systemic disease usually absent
   2. Is a primary glomerular disease in children
   3. In adults, can occur with a variety of systemic diseases
   4. 80% have minimal change disease on light microscopic examination, but 20% show histologic changes indicative of almost all forms of glomerulonephritis (prognosis in latter group is poor)
B. Incidence
   1. 1–3 cases per 100,000 children under 16 years
   2. Age group mostly affected is 1–7 years with peak incidence at 2–3 years
C. Etiology
   1. Unknown
   2. Pathogenesis not clear
   3. Occurs with Henoch-Schönlein disease, syphilis, malaria, tuberculosis, diabetes mellitus, amyloidosis, multiple myeloma, lupus erythematosis, sickle cell anemia, cyanotic congenital heart disease, renal vein thrombosis, drug toxicity, poison ivy, poison oak, bee sting (usually in adults)
   4. *Congenital nephrosis* appears before 6 months of age, is resistant to treatment, poor prognosis
D. Clinical and Laboratory Features
   1. Protineuria
   2. Edema
   3. Ascites
   4. Occasionally pleural effusion
   5. Malnutrition common
   6. Diarrhea common

7. Hematuria, if present, is usually minimal
8. Hypoproteinemia with hypoalbuminemia
9. Hypercholesterolemia
10. Reduced serum calcium (protein-bound fraction)
11. Elevated erythrocyte sedimentation rate

E. Course and Prognosis
1. Unusually susceptible to infections including pneumonia and peritonitis
2. Sepsis
3. Remissions and exacerbations may occur spontaneously
4. Survival rate 75% if intensively treated with corticosteroids

F. Treatment
1. Symptomatic
2. Appropriate antibiotic therapy for infections
3. Diuretics
4. Corticosteroid therapy has favorably influenced course of disease in most instances (treatment generally consists of 8-week course of steroid therapy)
5. Immunosuppressant or cytotoxic drugs (Cytoxan, methotrexate) if patient refractory or toxic to steroid therapy

HEMATURIA

A. Recurrent Hematuria
1. Recurrent episodes of hematuria that may extend over period of years
2. Acute episodes usually precipitated by viral infections
3. Between episodes, some have microscopic hematuria and mild to moderate proteinuria
4. Complete recovery occurs in many instances but long-term prognosis not established

B. Familial Benign Hematuria
1. Persistent hematuria with no incidence of deterioration in renal function
2. *Not* associated with hearing deficit
3. Transmitted as autosomal dominant

C. Hereditary Hematuria (Alport's Syndrome)
1. Associated with hearing loss and sometimes with cataracts
2. Clinical manifestations closely resemble those of acute glomerulonephritis
3. More severe in males
4. Renal disease and hearing loss both progressive, but not all develop renal insufficiency
5. No specific treatment for nephritis

D. Miscellaneous Causes
1. Abdominal trauma
2. Strenuous exercise
3. Jogging in males
4. Nephritis

5. Cystitis
6. Nephrolithiasis
7. Urinary tract tumors (including polyps)
8. Blood dyscrasias

HEMOLYTIC-UREMIC SYNDROME

A. Definition
    A syndrome characterized by nephropathy, anemia, thrombocytopenia
B. Etiology and Epidemiology
    1. Often preceded by viral infections, upper respiratory infections, gastroenteritis
    2. Occurs predominantly in Caucasians
    3. Most affected patients are children under 5 years of age
    4. Cause not identified
C. Clinical and Laboratory Features
    1. Abrupt onset following (within a week) flulike illness, gastroenteritis, or upper respiratory infection
    2. Signs and symptoms include pallor, purpura, easy bruising, irritability or lethargy, oliguria, jaundice, seizures, bloody diarrhea
    3. In mild cases, gradual improvement within 2-month period
    4. Severe cases characterized by progressive renal failure with hypertension
    5. Severe hemolytic anemia with anisocytosis, helmet-shaped cells, burr cells (red cells with protruding spikes)
D. Diagnosis
    1. Clinical manifestations (particularly hemolytic anemia, nephropathy, thrombocytopenia with acute onset following acute illness)
    2. Renal biopsy if necessary to exclude other renal conditions
E. Treatment
    1. Symptomatic
    2. Heparin, corticosteroids, cytotoxic agents, streptokinase have all been tried but no evidence that they are helpful
    3. No evidence that peritoneal dialysis reduces mortality but may be required for circulatory congestion
    4. Furosemide may also be useful to alleviate circulatory congestion
F. Prognosis
    1. Variable
    2. Recovery ranges from 15% to 60% depending on severity of disease

CRYPTORCHIDISM

A. Definition
    Undescended testis
B. Incidence

1. Vast majority of testes descend by first year of life
2. Spontaneous complete descent after infancy uncommon

C. Pathology
1. Right side more common
2. About 20% bilateral
3. Two types
   a. *Incomplete:* where testis stops somewhere along normal path
      1. Majority found in superficial inguinal canal
   b. *Ectopic testis:* present in abnormal location
      1. May be found in pubic, femoral, or perineal position
4. Associated with urinary tract anomalies

D. Manifestations
1. Absence of testis or testes from scrotum
2. Important to know that in childhood, cremasteric muscle can elevate testis out of scrotum in response to cold, stress, or palpation
   Careful examination demonstrates testis can be placed in scrotum
3. Cryptorchidism in genotypic male may present as hernia in phenotypic female (testicular feminization syndrome)

E. Diagnosis
Clinical signs

F. Complications
1. Torsion
2. Trauma
3. Malignancy

G. Treatment
1. Surgery at 5 years
2. Untreated cases have high incidence of malignancy and infertility

URINARY TRACT INFECTIONS

See Chapter 4, page 72.

BIBLIOGRAPHY

Hoekelman RA: Principles of Pediatrics. Health Care in the Young. New York, McGraw-Hill, 1978

Kaplan BS, Thomson PD, de Chadarevian JP: The hemolytic uremic syndrome. Pediatr Clin North Am 23:761–777, 1976

Lewy JE: Acute poststreptococcal glomerulonephritis. Pediatr Clin North Am 23:751–759, 1976

Margileth AM et al: Urinary tract bacterial injections. Office diagnosis and management. Pediatr Clin North Am 23:721–734, 1976

McDonald BM, McEnery PT: Glomerulonephritis in children. Clinical and morphologic characteristics and mechanisms of glomerular injury. Pediatr Clin North Am 23:691–706, 1976

Rance CP, Arbus GS, Balfe JW: Management of the nephrotic syndrome in children. Pediatr Clin North Am 23:735–750, 1976

Rudolph AM, Barnett HL, Einhorn WE: Pediatrics. New York, Appleton-Century-Crofts, 1977

Vaughan VC III, McKay RJ, Nelson WE: Nelson Textbook of Pediatrics. Philadelphia, W. B. Saunders, 1975

Pediatric
Hematology–Oncology

ANEMIAS (Fig. 68)

A. General Considerations
  1. Definition
    Reduction of hemoglobin and/or red blood cells below normal
  2. Pathogenesis
    a. May be caused by increased loss or destruction or decreased production of red blood cells
    b. Decreased production
      1. Genetic
      2. Decreased nutrition
      3. Decreased hormones
      4. Toxic drugs
      5. Neoplasms
    c. Increased loss or destruction
      1. Hemorrhage
      2. Genetic defect of enzyme, red cell membrane, hemoglobin
      3. Drugs

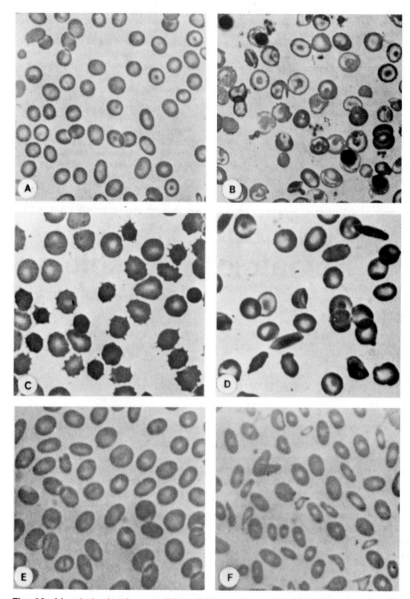

Fig. 68. Morphologic abnormalities of the red cell. **(A)** Thalassemia trait. **(B)** Thalassemia major. **(C)** Acanthocytes (abetalipoproteinemia). **(D)** Sickle cells (hemoglobin SS disease). **(E)** Elliptocytes (hereditary elliptocytosis). **(F)** Bizarre elliptocytes (hemolytic elliptocytosis). (*Pearson HA: In Vaughan VC III, McKay RJ, Nelson WE (eds): Nelson Textbook of Pediatrics, p 1121. Philadelphia, W. B. Saunders, 1975*)

3. Morphology
   a. Normocytic, normochromic
      1. Hemorrhage
      2. Hemolytic anemia
      3. Miscellaneous
   b. Microcytic, hypochromic
      1. Iron deficiency
      2. Lead poisoning
      3. Thalassemia
      4. Pyridoxine (vitamin B$_6$) deficiency
      5. Sideroblastic anemia*
   c. Macrocytic, normochromic
      1. Pernicious anemia
      2. Folic acid deficiency
      3. Drugs
      4. Bone marrow failure
      5. Neoplasms
4. Manifestations
   a. Fatigue, pallor, jaundice, dyspnea on exertion, vertigo, dizziness, orthopnea, menstrual irregularities
   b. Sometimes splenomegaly, hepatomegaly, pale mucous membranes, tachycardia, bruits, decreased diastolic blood pressure
5. Diagnosis
   a. Signs and symptoms
      Detailed nutritional and family histories should be done
   b. Complete blood count
   c. Bone marrow aspiration and biopsy occasionally necessary
6. Treatment
   Depends on type of anemia
B. Iron Deficiency Anemia
   1. Incidence
      a. Most common nutritional deficiency in pediatric patients
      b. Particularly in formula-fed infants (bioavailability of iron greater in breast milk than cow's milk)
   2. Etiology
      a. Inadequate intake
      b. Blood loss
         About one-third of infants with iron deficiency have guaiac-positive stools
   3. Manifestations
      a. Pallor (key finding)
      b. Tachycardia, murmurs, splenomegaly may occur
      c. Saturation of iron-binding protein less than 15%

* See Glossary

      d. Hypochromic microcytic anemia

      e. Reticulocytes normal or slightly elevated

      f. Decreased iron in bone marrow (Prussian blue stain)

   4. Diagnosis

      a. Clinical signs and symptoms

      b. Bone marrow examination

      c. Response to iron therapy

   5. Complications

      Congestive heart failure

   6. Treatment

      a. Oral ferrous salts (sulfate, gluconate) for 4–6 weeks after normal blood indices are attained

      b. Restrict milk since large intake may decrease absorption of iron

      c. Parenteral iron therapy infrequently used

      d. Transfusion rarely indicated because of prompt response to therapy

      e. Reticulocytosis seen 72–96 hours after therapy started, then hemoglobin rises

      f. *Prophylaxis:* Formula-fed infants should have supplemental iron until 1 year of age

C. Megaloblastic Anemia

   1. Definition

      Anemia accompanied by enlarged peripheral red blood cells (macrocytes). Bone marrow shows enlarged precursor red blood cells with abnormal mitotic figures and nuclear fragments (megaloblasts)

   2. Pathogenesis

      a. Nutritional deficiency causes slowing of DNA synthesis. RNA synthesis occurs at same rate, which means that cytoplasm matures faster than nucleus

      b. Nutritional deficiencies that cause megaloblastic anemia

         1. Vitamin B_{12} (pernicious anemia)

         2. Folic acid

         3. Ascorbic acid, tocopherol (vitamin E), thiamine (rare)

      c. Drug-induced megaloblastic anemia

         Hydantoin

         Thought to cause folic acid deficiency

   3. Folic acid deficiency

      a. Caused by inadequate intake, by drugs inhibiting its absorption or utilization, decreased absorption (malabsorption), increased requirement, increased excretion

      b. Folate requirement increased in malignant disease, hyperthyroidism, hemolytic disorders

      c. Is most common cause of megaloblastic anemia of infancy

      d. Manifestations

         1. Peak incidence at about 4–7 months

         2. Symptoms of anemia plus irritability, failure to gain weight, chronic diarrhea. May have signs of scurvy (vitamin C deficiency)

3. Peripheral blood shows low reticulocyte count, macrocytes, large nucleated red blood cells, hypersegmented neutrophils (4 or more lobes in nucleus), neutropenia and thrombocytopenia, high mean corpuscular volume (MCV)
4. Decreased serum folic acid
5. Bone marrow hypercellularity with megaloblasts

e. Diagnosis
   1. Clinical signs and symptoms
   2. Peripheral blood hemogram
   3. Bone marrow aspirate and biopsy
   4. Serum folic acid and vitamin B_{12} determinations

f. Treatment
   1. Folic acid, orally or parenterally
   2. Treat underlying disorder if present
   3. Transfusion if patient severely ill or anemic
   4. Response to therapy should begin in about 72 hours

4. Vitamin B_{12} deficiency (pernicious anemia)
   a. Absorption of B_{12} dependent upon binding with glycoprotein (intrinsic factor) secreted in stomach
   b. Causes of deficiency
      1. Inadequate intake (diet)
      2. Abnormal absorption
         a. Decreased or absent intrinsic factor
         b. Failure of absorption in small intestine
            i. Secondary to intestinal disease (Crohn's disease)
            ii. Specific B_{12} malabsorption (as with use of chelating agents)
            iii. Competition for B_{12} [blind intestinal loops, fistulas, *Diphyllobothrium latum* (tapeworm)]
      3. Defective transport
      4. Abnormal metabolism
   c. Clinical manifestations
      1. Usually occurs during first 2 years of life
      2. Signs and symptoms of anemia plus reddened sore tongue, paresthesias,* ataxia, hyporeflexia, positive Babinski sign, clonus, coma, pigmentation of skin
      3. Laboratory findings as described for folic acid deficiency
      4. Decreased serum vitamin B_{12}
   d. Diagnosis
      1. Clinical signs and symptoms
      2. Peripheral blood hemogram
      3. Bone marrow aspirate and biopsy
      4. Serum folic acid and vitamin B_{12} determinations
      5. Schilling test*

* See Glossary

  e. Treatment
    1. Usually requires lifelong treatment
    2. Parenteral vitamin B_{12}
    3. Treat underlying condition if present
    4. Transfusion if severely ill or severely anemic
D. Lead Poisoning
  1. Seen primarily in young children
  2. Manifestations
    a. Hyperirritability, anorexia, fatigue, vomiting, constipation, abdominal pain
    b. May develop vomiting, ataxia, altered consciousness, coma, seizures (acute encephalopathy)
        Most common in summer months (in children 1–3 years of age)
    c. Anemia (microcytic hypochromic with basophilic stippling of red blood cells)
  3. Diagnosis
    a. Clinical signs and symptoms
    b. Peripheral blood hemogram
    c. Serum lead level
  4. Complications
    a. Seizure disorders
    b. Hyperkinetic conditions
    c. Mental impairment
    d. Peripheral neuropathy (rare in children)
  5. Treatment
    a. Removal of lead sources
    b. Parenteral calcium EDTA
    c. If signs of acute encephalopathy present, use calcium EDTA and BAL in combined regimen
    d. Appropriate fluid and electrolyte management
E. Defects of Marrow
  1. Congenital hypoplastic anemia (Diamond-Blackfan syndrome)
    a. Pure red cell hypoplasia
    b. Other congenital anomalies commonly present
    c. Pallor is only symptom
    d. Require chronic transfusions
    e. Treat with corticosteroids
  2. Numerous drugs or infections can cause selective red cell hypoplasia or panhypoplasia
F. Hemolytic Anemias
  1. Hereditary spherocytosis
    a. Definition
        Anemia caused by red cell membrane defect manifested microscopically by loss of cellular central pallor (characteristic of biconcave disc shape of red blood cell)
    b. Incidence and genetics

       1. 1 in 5000

       2. Autosomal dominant

       3. Sporadic cases reported

  c. Manifestations

       1. Symptoms variable depending on severity of defect

       2. Onset usually in infancy

       3. Slight jaundice, anemia, splenomegaly

       4. Gallstones in older children and adolescents

       5. Peripheral blood shows reticulocytosis, spherocytes, anemia, hyper-bilirubinemia

       6. Immersion in hypotonic saline causes higher hemolytic rate than normal cells

  d. Diagnosis

       1. Clinical signs and symptoms

       2. Peripheral blood hemogram

       3. Serum bilirubin

       4. Hypotonic saline test

  e. Complications

      Aplastic crisis

         Acute reticulocytopenia secondary to infection

  f. Treatment

       1. Splenectomy treatment of choice

          a. Prolongs red cell life span

          b. Optimum age for surgery is 5 years

       2. Transfusions for anemia and hypoplastic crisis

          a. Usually not needed after surgery

2. Hereditary elliptocytosis

  a. Definition

      Anemia caused by defect of red blood cell membrane characterized by oval red blood cells in peripheral smear

  b. Incidence and genetics

       1. 1 in 2500

       2. Significant anemia in about 10% of patients

       3. Autosomal dominant

  c. Clinical manifestations

       1. Most patients asymptomatic

       2. Anemic patients' signs and symptoms similar to those of patients with spherocytosis

       3. Peripheral smear shows elliptocytes

       4. Laboratory tests of symptomatic patients similar to those of patients with spherocytosis

  d. Diagnosis

      As described for spherocytosis

  e. Complications

      Hypoplastic crisis

    f. Treatment
       1. Transfusions
       2. Splenectomy treatment of choice if symptomatic
  3. Paroxysmal nocturnal hemoglobinuria (PNH)
    a. Definition
       1. Rare illness manifested by episodes of nighttime hemoglobinuria (caused by hemolysis within renal parenchyma)
       2. Frequently, hemolysis may be chronic and occur anytime (day or night)
       3. Hemolysis thought to be secondary to membrane defect
    b. Manifestations
       1. About 20% of patients have hemoglobinuria
       2. Fatigue, pallor, other symptoms of anemia are presenting complaints
       3. Can be mild or severe
       4. Peripheral blood shows hypochromia and microcytosis if hemolysis severe and chronic
       5. Leukopenia often present
       6. Bone marrow shows erythrohyperplasia
       7. Hemoglobin and hemosiderin in urine
       8. Immersion of blood in acid solution (Ham test) or in isotonic sucrose causes hemolysis
    c. Diagnosis
       1. Clinical signs and symptoms
       2. Peripheral blood hemogram
       3. Urine for hemoglobin and hemosiderin
       4. Sugar water and Ham test
    d. Complications
       1. Infection
       2. Hemorrhage
       3. Thrombosis
          About 50% of patients die from this complication
    e. Treatment
       1. No definitive treatment
       2. Transfusion for severe anemia
  4. Glucose-6-phosphate dehydrogenase (G6PD) deficiency
    a. General considerations
       1. Characterized by episodic or chronic hemolytic anemia caused by infection or drugs
       2. X-linked recessive
          Heterozygotic females usually unaffected
       3. Non-Mediterranean Caucasians least affected
       4. Older red blood cells deficient in enzyme
    b. Manifestations
       1. Drug- or infection-induced hemolytic anemia
          a. Hemolysis begins 48–96 hours after taking oxidant drug (sulfonamides, antipyretics, antimalarial agents)
          b. Pallor, jaundice, hemoglobinuria (dark urine), back pain

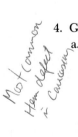

Most common Hem defect in Caucasian

    c. In severe cases, shock, cardiovascular collapse, death

   2. Chronic hemolytic anemia

    a. Chronic anemia and jaundice

    b. Oxidant drugs aggravate condition

  c. Diagnosis

   1. Quantitative measurement of G6PD

    Should not be done immediately after hemolytic episode because G6PD becomes falsely elevated due to abundance of young erythrocytes

   2. Clinical signs and symptoms

  d. Complications

   1. Shock

   2. Death

  e. Treatment

   1. Identification of population at risk

    Careful avoidance of oxidant drugs

   2. Transfusion for acute episode

   3. Splenectomy may lessen severity

    Not effective in chronic hemolytic anemia

G. Sickle Cell Disease

 1. General considerations

  a. Chronic hemolytic anemia due to abnormal hemoglobin structure

  b. Abnormal hemoglobin caused by substitution of valine for glutamic acid in number 6 position of beta polypeptide chain

  c. Sickle cell anemia is homozygous state

 2. Incidence

  In blacks, Mediterranean Caucasians

 3. Manifestations

  a. Appears late in first year (after fetal hemoglobin disappears)

  b. Undergo several types of crises

   1. Vaso-occlusive crisis: Due to occlusion of small vessels. May be preceded by infection

    a. Infants develop painful swelling of hands and feet (hand-foot syndrome). May be first presentation of disease

    b. Roentgenogram shows bone destruction

    c. Also acute abdominal pain, strokes, pulmonary infarction

   2. Sequestration crisis: Liver and spleen pool large amounts of blood. Develop signs of circulatory collapse

   3. Aplastic crisis: Occurs because of drop in marrow production of erythrocytes. Usually preceded by infection

   4. Hyperhemolytic crisis: Unusual, occurs when sickle cell patient is also G6PD deficient and takes oxidant drug. Manifested by jaundice, anemia, reticulocytosis

  c. Hemoglobin about 6–8 g/dl, reticulocyte count about 10%, peripheral smear shows hypochromia, sickled cells, white blood cells 15,000–25,000

 4. Diagnosis

a. Clinical signs and symptoms
b. Serum electrophoresis
c. Sickle cell test (deoxygenating erythrocytes and then viewing sickle-shaped cells microscopically)
5. Complications
   a. Progressive impairment of liver function
   b. Gallstones
   c. Impaired renal function
   d. Autosplenectomy (due to multiple infarcts)
   e. Increased susceptibility to pneumococcus, H. influenzae, meningococcus
   f. Osteomyelitis (especially salmonella)
6. Treatment
   For crisis
   1. Analgesics
   2. Keep patient well hydrated to prevent sickling
   3. Transfusions when lungs or central nervous system extensively involved
H. Sickle Cell Trait
  1. Patient heterozygous (HS) for sickle cell
  2. Usually asymptomatic
  3. Renal infarcts promoted by changes in pH, oxygenation, and ionic concentration around loop of Henle
   a. Most sickle cell trait patients have impaired urinary concentration
   b. Hematuria not infrequent
  4. Splenic infarction in patients flying in unpressurized aircraft at high altitudes
I. Thalassemia
  1. General considerations
   a. Hereditary anemia caused by deficient synthesis of hemoglobin polypeptide chains
   b. Anemia is hypochromic, microcytic
   c. Occurs primarily in blacks, Orientals, Mediterraneans, and Caucasions
   d. Many different genes can cause decrease of beta chain synthesis
     Genes vary in severity from no synthesis of beta chain to slightly decreased synthesis
  2. Homozygous alpha thalassemia (thalassemia major)
   a. Lethal condition causing stillbirth or neonatal death
   b. Generalized edema in neonate (hydrops fetalis)
   c. Patient cannot produce fetal or adult hemoglobin because no alpha chains
   d. Marked predominance of gamma chain hemoglobin (Bart's hemoglobin)
  3. Heterozygous alpha thalassemia (thalassemia minor)
   Two forms
   1. Silent carrier
    a. Slight reduction of alpha chain synthesis
    b. Asymptomatic
   2. Alpha thalassemia trait
    a. Moderate reduction of alpha chain synthesis

   b. Mild anemia

   c. Family history of anemia or stillbirth

   d. Significant amount of Bart's hemoglobin present at birth (about 5%)

   e. Most prominent in Orientals, but can occur in blacks

4. Homozygous beta thalassemia (thalassemia major, Cooley's anemia)

 a. General considerations

   1. About 10% have no beta chain synthesis

   2. Can have persistent elevated fetal hemoglobin

     Disease course similar to that of heterozygous form

   3. Fetal hemoglobin production insufficient

   4. Prevalent in Mediterraneans and Orientals

 b. Clinical manifestations

   1. No anemia in neonatal period

   2. Anemia begins during first few months of life, is progressive and severe

   3. Pallor, icterus, hepatosplenomegaly, poor feeding

   4. Periodic fever, diarrhea

   5. Later, child is small for age but head may appear large, mongoloid facies, thickened skull bones, mild jaundice, cardiomegaly

   6. Peripheral blood shows nucleated erythrocytes, reticulocytosis, hypochromia, microcytosis, leukocytosis, hemoglobin generally below 8 g/dl

   7. Roentgenogram of skull shows thickened diploë with "hair on end" appearance of bone spicules (Fig. 69)

 c. Diagnosis

   1. Clinical signs and symptoms

   2. Peripheral blood hemogram

   3. Skull roentgenogram

   4. Serum electrophoresis

 d. Complications

   1. Hemosiderosis (secondary to multiple transfusions)

    a. Diabetes mellitus (secondary to pancreatic damage)

    b. Cardiac and hepatic damage

   2. Pericarditis

   3. Congestive heart failure

   4. Death (usually in second decade)

 e. Treatment

   1. Blood transfusion

    a. Only given to maintain level of 9–10 g/dl

    b. Should be started early in life (about 4–6 years)

    c. Use of iron chelating agents (*i.e.*, deferoxamine, EDTA) to prevent hemosiderosis is of questionable value

   2. Splenectomy

    a. Advised when anemia develops rapidly after transfusion, with severe thrombocytopenia, or with marked splenomegaly

    b. Risks include increased susceptibility to sepsis

5. Heterozygous beta thalassemia (thalassemia minor)

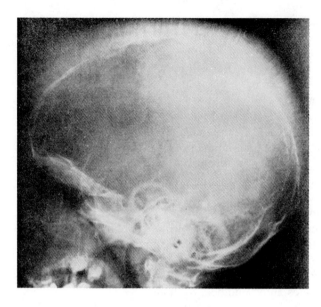

Fig. 69. Thalassemia major. Roentgenogram of skull showing overgrowth of the maxilla with opacification of the sinuses. The diploic spaces are widened, with prominent vertical trabeculae (hair on end). (*Pearson HA: In Vaughan VC III, McKay RJ, Nelson W (eds): Nelson Textbook of Pediatrics, p 1128. Philadelphia, W. B. Saunders, 1975*)

   a. General considerations

      Many different forms varying from asymptomatic carrier to moderate anemia. Prevalent in Mediterraneans

   b. Manifestations

      1. Mild anemia mimicking iron deficiency (often only symptom)

      2. Splenomegaly may be present

      3. Family history of stillborns or anemia

      4. Occasionally symptoms similar to homozygous state

      5. Mean corpuscular volume and mean corpuscular hemoglobin decreased, hemoglobin slightly decreased or normal

   c. Diagnosis

      1. Clinical signs and symptoms

      2. Serum electrophoresis

   d. Treatment

      Therapy depends on severity of symptoms

ANAPHYLACTOID PURPURA (HENOCH-SCHÖNLEIN)

A. Definition

   Acquired disease of unknown etiology manifested by nonthrombocytopenic purpura, various joint and visceral abnormalities with diffuse vasculitis

B. Incidence

   1. Patients 6 months–16 years most often affected

   2. Males most often involved

   3. Occurs primarily in spring and fall

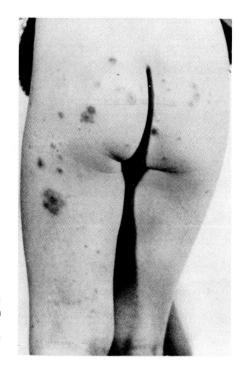

Fig. 70. Early eruption of Henoch-Schoenlein syndrome showing urticarial lesions, some with central areas of hemorrhage. (*Silber DL: Henoch-Schoenlein Syndrome. Pediatr Clin North Am 19:1061, 1972*)

C. Etiology

    Thought to be immune response to antigen (infection, vaccine, insect bite, antibiotic)

D. Manifestations

    1. Symmetric purpura involving primarily buttocks and lower extremities associated with maculopapular rash (Fig. 70)

    2. Purpura may involve extensor surface of arms, palms, soles, or genitalia

       Trunk almost always spared

    3. Edema, arthritis (usually knees and ankles)

    4. Gastrointestinal tract and kidneys most often involved

       a. Abdominal pain, nausea, vomiting, bloody stools

       b. Hematuria, casts, proteinuria

    5. Central nervous system involvement uncommon

E. Diagnosis

    1. Clinical signs and symptoms

    2. Observation to determine hemostatic function and visceral involvement

       a. Platelet count, prothrombin time, partial thromboplastin time, hematocrit

       b. Stool guaiac, urinalysis, serum creatinine

F. Complications

    1. Bowel perforation

    2. Intussusception

    3. Chronic glomerulonephritis

    4. Renal failure

    5. Subarachnoid hemorrhage

    6. Death (less than 5%)

G. Treatment

    1. Analgesics

       Acetaminophen

    2. Corticosteroids (only for moderate or severe symptoms)

       a. Improve edema, arthralgia, and abdominal pain

       b. No beneficial effects on purpura or renal lesions

H. Prognosis

    1. Majority of cases have only one episode

    2. Some have periodic episodes for 2–3 years, then permanent cure

THROMBOCYTOPENIA

A. General Considerations

    1. Definition

       Decrease in serum platelets

    2. Types

       a. Acquired thrombocytopenia

          1. Increased destruction or loss of platelets

             a. Idiopathic thrombocytopenic purpura

             b. Immunologic disorder

             c. Infections

          2. Decreased or defective production of platelets

             a. Aplastic anemia (bone marrow aplasia secondary to drugs, infections, idiopathic)

             b. Malignant invasion of marrow

       b. Inherited thrombocytopenic purpura

          1. Decreased production

             a. *Fanconi's anemia:* Pancytopenia associated with various congenital anomalies

             b. Thrombocytopenia with absent radius (*TAR syndrome*)

          2. Increased destruction

             Wiskott-Aldrich syndrome: Rare sex-linked recessive disease manifested by chronic thrombocytopenia, eczema, recurrent infections

B. Idiopathic Thrombocytopenic Purpura (ITP)

    1. Definition

       a. Coagulation disorder manifested by acute, recurrent, or chronic thrombocytopenic purpura in absence of other identifiable types of thrombocytopenia

       b. Types

          1. *Acute:* Complete remission within 6 months

    2. Chronic: Complete remission not achieved within 6 months
2. Incidence
   a. Children and young adults affected most
   b. Acute form seen in young children
   c. Chronic form more common in older children and adults
3. Etiology
   a. Exact etiology unknown
   b. Known to be immunologic condition where patient's antibodies are directed against platelets
4. Manifestations
   a. Purpura varying from petechiae to large ecchymotic areas in random distribution
   b. Epistaxis, bloody stools, hematuria (uncommon)
   c. *No* lymphadenopathy or hepatosplenomegaly
   d. History of preceding illness in acute form
   e. Insidious onset in chronic form
   f. Peripheral blood shows decreased platelets
   g. Anemia may be present
   h. Marrow shows abundance of megakaryocytes
5. Diagnosis
   a. Clinical signs and symptoms
   b. Peripheral blood smear and platelet count
   c. Bone marrow aspirate and biopsy
6. Complications
   a. Intracranial hemorrhage (infrequent)
   b. Death (rare)
7. Treatment
   a. Acute
      1. *Supportive:* Replace acute blood loss if marked, ferrous sulfate supplement, follow patient's course
      2. *Corticosteroids:* If threat of intracranial hemorrhage present or symptoms marked
         Steroids thought to stabilize capillary walls but do not affect platelet destruction
      3. *Splenectomy:* Only if life-threatening hemorrhage present
   b. Chronic
      1. Chronic steroid therapy to be avoided
      2. Elective splenectomy (1 year after onset of disease may be beneficial)
      3. Immunosuppressive therapy only if splenectomy fails to achieve remission
8. Prognosis
   Acute
      1. About 80–90% of young children make complete recovery
      2. Some patients have underlying disease that is later diagnosed
      3. About 5% progress to chronic form

COAGULATION DEFECTS

Hemophilia
1. Definition
   Severe hemorrhagic disease of males caused by hereditary deficiency of factors VIII, IX, and XI
2. Classic hemophilia (factor VIII deficiency)
   a. Incidence and genetics
      1. Most common hereditary coagulation disorder
      2. 1 in 10,000 white male births
      3. X-linked recessive trait
   b. Manifestations
      1. Recognized shortly after birth (usually intense hemorrhage after circumcision)
      2. Significant hemorrhage may not occur until patient begins walking
      3. Frequently develop bleeding into joint spaces (hemarthroses), particularly of knees, ankles, elbows
      4. Hematuria, oral bleeding, bloody stools, epistaxis also occurs
      5. Prolonged PTT, with normal PT, platelet count, and function
   c. Diagnosis
      1. Clinical signs and symptoms
      2. PTT, PT, platelet count and function, factor VIII assay
   d. Complications
      1. Degenerative arthritis
      2. Intracranial bleeding (major cause of death)
      3. Intraspinal hemorrhage (infrequent)
      4. Peripheral nerve hemorrhage
      5. Marked blood loss
   e. Treatment
      1. Hemarthrosis
         a. Cold compresses
         b. Analgesics (*not aspirin*, because aspirin causes platelat dysfunction and may aggravate the disorder)
         c. Aspiration of involved joint (if hemorrhage severe)
         d. Factor VIII transfusions
      2. Severe life-threatening hemorrhage
         Large factor VIII transfusion
      3. Hematuria
         a. Steroids, if hematuria not associated with trauma
         b. Usually not responsive to factor VIII transfusion
      4. Oral bleeding
         a. Aminocaproic acid orally
         b. Factor VIII transfusion
         c. Topical thrombin

3. Christmas disease (factor IX deficiency, hemophilia B)
   a. Incidence and genetics
      1. Constitutes about 15% of all hemophilias
      2. X-linked recessive
   b. Manifestations
      1. Identical to classic hemophilia
      2. Laboratory data same, except that deficiency is of factor IX
   c. Diagnosis
      1. Clinical signs and symptoms
      2. PT, PTT, platelet count and function, factor IX assay
   d. Complications and treatment
      Essentially same as for classic hemophilia
4. Factor XI deficiency
   Rare
5. Von Willebrand's disease
   a. Definition
      Hemorrhagic disorder of males and females caused by factor VIII deficiency plus platelet dysfunction
   b. Incidence and genetics
      1. Ranks third in frequency of inherited coagulation disorders (behind classic hemophilia and Christmas disease)
      2. Autosomal dominant
   c. Manifestations
      1. Mucocutaneous bleeding, epistaxis, bleeding from gums, prolonged ooz- of minor lacerations
      2. Prolonged bleeding time and PTT, deficient platelet adhesion to glass beads, decreased factor VIII
   d. Diagnosis
      1. Clinical signs and symptoms
      2. Bleeding time, PT, PTT, platelet function studies, assay for factor VIII
   e. Complications
      Appreciable blood loss
   f. Treatment
      1. Factor VIII for severe hemorrhage
      2. Local hemostatic treatment usually effective
6. Disseminated intravascular coagulation (DIC)
   a. Definition
      Acquired coagulation disorder associated with underlying disease caused by uncontrolled coagulation and fibrinolysis
   b. Incidence and etiology
      1. Life-threatening DIC rare in childhood
      2. Milder forms common
      3. Seen with variety of diseases
      4. Exact etiology unknown

     5. Begins with thrombotic process, then hemorrhage secondary to consumption of clotting factors

  c. Manifestations

     1. Hemorrhage (not ischemia) dominant clinical finding

     2. Purpura (ecchymotic), anemia, various degrees of circulatory failure

     3. Symptoms associated with underlying disease

     4. Decreased platelets, prolonged PT, PTT, fibrin-split products and prolonged thrombin clotting time (TCT), with decrease in factors I, II, V, VIII

  d. Diagnosis

     1. Clinical signs and symptoms

     2. PT, PTT, TCT, platelet count, fibrin-split products, assay for factors V and VIII

  e. Complications

     1. Shock

     2. Major hemorrhage

     3. Organ necrosis

  f. Treatment

     1. Treat underlying condition

     2. Supportive care

     3. Fresh whole plasma and platelet transfusions if active bleeding

     4. Heparin therapy if no improvement (basic disease process is *thrombosis*—controversial)

LEUKEMIA

A. Definition

  1. Malignancy of blood-forming organs

  2. Most common form of malignancy in childhood

B. Acute Lymphocytic Leukemia

  1. Incidence

     Most common form of childhood leukemia

  2. Cell type

     a. Lymphocyte surface markers can designate whether tumors are B cells, T cells, or null cells (no markers)

     b. Majority are null cells

  3. Manifestations

     a. Fever, bleeding, hepatosplenomegaly, lymphadenopathy

     b. May present with joint pains, pallor, slow healing, recurrent infections

     c. Peripheral blood studies may show lymphoblasts

     d. Bone marrow shows many lymphoblasts

  4. Diagnosis

     a. Clinical signs and symptoms

     b. Peripheral blood hemogram

    c. Bone marrow aspirate and biopsy
    d. Immunologic surface markers
5. Complications
    a. Hyperuricemia
        Can lead to renal failure
    b. Hypercalcemia or hypocalcemia
    c. Hemorrhage
    d. Infection
        1. Bacterial: Pseudomonas aeruginosa, Staphylococcus aureus, Hemophilus influenzae, Proteus mirabilis
        2. Fungal: Candida albicans, Aspergillus species, Cryptococcus neoformans
        3. Protozoan: Pneumocystis carinii
        4. Viral: Varicella-zoster, cytomegalovirus, herpes simplex
6. Central nervous system and extramedullary leukemia
    a. Meningeal involvement
        1. Frequent site for relapse
        2. May develop various neurologic signs and symptoms
        3. Presence of high leukocyte count increases likelihood of meningeal disease
        4. Diagnosis by lumbar puncture
    b. Testicular disease
        1. Can be seen in primary disease
        2. Significant site for relapse
        3. Presence of small nests of leukemic cells can herald relapse despite rest of body being disease free
        4. Must continually be evaluated clinically
        5. Diagnosis by clinical signs and symptoms and by testicular biopsy
    c. Leukemic infiltration can occur in many organs
        1. Usually seen in widespread disease
        2. Can occur in single organ, heralding relapse
    d. Diagnosis of relapse
        1. Clinical signs and symptoms
        2. Bone marrow aspirate and biopsy
            Greater than 5% lymphoblasts constitutes relapse
        3. Lumbar puncture
            Greater than 5 leukemic cells/cu mm with atraumatic tap
        4. Testicular biopsy
7. Prognosis
    a. Better prognosis
        1. Age 3–6 years
        2. Peripheral leukocyte count less than 10,000/cu mm
        3. Null cell markers (not firmly established)
        4. Greater than 85% remain in remission three years after diagnosis
    b. Poor prognosis
        1. Leukocyte count greater than 50,000/cu mm

2. Age less than 3 years, greater than 7 years
3. B- or T-cell markers
4. Meningeal involvement
5. Less than 50% in remission two years after diagnosis

8. Treatment
   a. Experimental
   b. All patients receive intrathecal methotrexate and cranial irradiation to prevent central nervous system relapse
   c. Patients receive differing amounts of chemotherapy depending on presenting clinical findings and treatment protocol

C. Acute Myelogenous Leukemia
   1. Tumor composed of immature myeloid cells
   2. Infrequently occurs in children
   3. Symptoms similar to those of lymphocytic leukemia
   4. Infections may dominate clinical picture
   5. Poorer prognosis than acute lymphocytic leukemia
   6. Treatment experimental

LYMPHOMAS

A. Definition
   Malignancy of lymphoid tissue
B. Hodgkin's Disease
   1. Incidence
      a. Rare before 2 years of age
      b. About 10% of patients with Hodgkin's disease are 15 years or less
      c. Seen more frequently in males
      d. Disease incidence peaks at 20 and at 60 years
   2. Histology
      a. Four different microscopic types
         1. *Lymphocyte predominant:* Node replaced by large numbers of monotonous appearing lymphocytes
         2. *Mixed cellularity:* Node contains lymphocytes, neutrophils, eosinophils, histiocytes, plasma cells
         3. *Lymphocyte depleted:* Node may be mostly fibrotic, containing few cells, or may have many anaplastic cells
         4. *Nodular sclerosis:* Bands of collagen enclosing nodules of abnormal lymphocytes
      b. Large multinucleated cells, often binucleated (Reed-Sternberg cells), present in all histologic types
         Reed-Sternberg cells essential for diagnosis of Hodgkin's disease
   3. Manifestations
      a. Nontender lymphadenopathy, may have history of rapid or slow enlargement

    b. Fever, night sweats, weight loss may be present

    c. Hepatosplenomegaly sometimes present

    d. Laboratory tests may reveal anemia or elevated sedimentation rate

  4. Diagnosis

    a. Clinical signs and symptoms

    b. Biopsy of enlarged node

  5. Determining extent of disease (staging)

    a. Chest roentgenogram, intravenous pyelogram, lymphangiogram

    b. Peripheral hemogram, urinalysis, liver function tests

    c. Liver–spleen scan

    d. Laparotomy including splenectomy, multiple node biopsies, liver biopsy

    e. Stages

      1. *Stage I:* One lymph node region involved

      2. *Stage II:* Two or more lymph node regions involved above or below diaphragm

      3. *Stage III:* Lymphoma on both sides of diaphragm involved

      4. *Stage IV:* Extralymphoreticular system involved

  6. Prognosis

    a. *Good prognosis:* Stage I or II, absence of night sweats and fever, histologic picture of nodular sclerosis or lymphocyte predominance

    b. *Poor prognosis:* Stage III or IV, presence of night sweats and fever, histologic picture of lymphocyte depletion

    c. Overall prognosis in childhood is good

  7. Complications

    a. Infection

    b. Superior vena cava obstruction

  8. Treatment

    a. Tumor highly sensitive to radiation

    b. Various radiation field patterns used depending on lymph regions involved and stage of disease

    c. Chemotherapy used in conjunction with radiotherapy, depending on stage of disease

C. Non-Hodgkin's Lymphoma

  1. Incidence

    a. Highest in 15- to 35-year-old group

    b. Next most commonly seen in children under 15 years

    c. Males most commonly involved

  2. Histology

    a. Abnormal, monotonous appearance of lymphocytes

    b. Reed-Sternberg cells not present

  3. Manifestations

    a. Painless, nontender lymphadenopathy

    b. Weight loss, fever, anorexia may be present

    c. Hepatic and splenic involvement frequently seen

    d. Patient usually presents with widespread disease (stage III or IV)

4. Diagnosis and staging
   Same as for Hodgkin's disease
5. Prognosis
   Poorer than Hodgkin's disease
6. Complications
   a. Infection
   b. Superior vena cava obstruction
   c. Leukemic transformation
   d. Central nervous system involvement
7. Treatment
   Combination radiotherapy and chemotherapy

NEUROBLASTOMA (Figs. 71, 72)

A. Definition
   1. Malignant tumor arising from sympathetic ganglion precursor cells
   2. *Sites* include adrenal medulla, sympathetic chain (abdomen, thorax, pelvis), para-aortic sympathetic bodies of Zuckerkandl
B. Incidence
   1. Seen mainly in infancy (about 70% recognized under 4 years of age)
   2. Slightly more common in females
   3. Second or third most frequent cause of abdominal mass in neonate
C. Histology
   1. Cellular mass of small basophilic cells
   2. Presence of pseudorosettes distinguishing trademark
D. Metastatic Spread
   1. Spreads by direct extension or hematogenous seeding
   2. Most common distant organs involved are liver, bones, lungs
E. Manifestations
   1. Depends on primary site
   2. Adrenal gland
      a. Abdominal mass, malaise, anorexia, fever
      b. Bone pain and fever may mimic rheumatic fever
   3. Thorax
      Asymptomatic usually but can have cough and chest pain
   4. Pelvis
      Bowel complaints, lumbar pain, rectal pain
   5. Abdominal roentgenogram may show lateral displacement of ureter ("drooping lily" effect) and/or stippled calcification of adrenal gland
   6. Urine shows elevated vanilmandelic acid (VMA) and/or homovanillic acid (HVA) in about 75% of cases
F. Diagnosis
   1. Clinical signs and symptoms
   2. Abdominal films

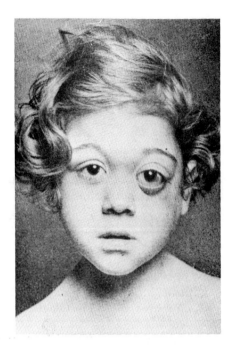

Fig. 71. Proptosis with subconjunctival and periorbital hemorrhage as the presenting feature of adrenal neuroblastoma. (*Hutchison JH: Practical Paediatric Problems. Lloyd-Luke Publication, p 216. Chicago, Year Book (distributor), 1975*)

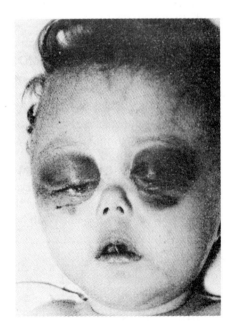

Fig. 72. Gross proptosis and periorbital ecchymosis in late stage of illness from neuroblastoma. (*Hutchison JH: Practical Paediatric Problems, p 216. Lloyd-Luke Publication. Chicago, Year Book (distributor) 1975*)

    3. Urine analysis for VMA
    4. Biopsy
G. Staging
        Studies for staging include:
        a. Bone marrow aspirate
        b. Peripheral hemogram
        c. Skeletal survey
        d. Liver–spleen scan
        e. Liver function tests
        f. Stages
            1. *Stage I:* Tumor totally within organ
            2. *Stage II:* Tumor spread outside organ but not crossing midline
            3. *Stage III:* Tumor spread across midline
            4. *Stage IV:* Tumor spread to distant organs
H. Prognosis
    1. *Better prognosis:* Early age at diagnosis (less than 2 years), stage I or II, presence of mature ganglion cells on microscopic examination
    2. *Poor prognosis:* Older age at diagnosis (greater than 2 years), stage III or IV, primitive cells on histologic examination
 I. Treatment
    1. Surgery
    2. Chemotherapy
    3. Radiotherapy

WILMS' TUMOR (NEPHROBLASTOMA)

A. Definition
        Malignant primitive neoplasm of kidneys
B. Incidence and Associated Conditions
    1. Occurs most often in young child
    2. Second or third most frequent cause of abdominal mass in neonate
    3. About 50% of cases diagnosed before 3 years of age
    4. Equal incidence in boys and girls
    5. Bilateral involvement in less than 10% of cases
    6. Associated with congenital heart disease, aniridia, horseshoe kidney, cryptorchidism
C. Manifestations
    1. Abdominal mass, pain, fever, hematuria
    2. Roentgenographic demonstration of mass that may be calcified
D. Diagnosis
    1. Clinical signs and symptoms
    2. Abdominal film, intravenous pyelogram
    3. Urinalysis
E. Staging
        Similar to neuroblastoma

F. Prognosis
    1. *Better prognosis:* Under 2 years of age at diagnosis, stage I
    2. *Poor prognosis:* Greater than 2 years of age, stage III or IV
G. Treatment
    1. Surgery
    2. Chemotherapy
    3. Radiotherapy

BONE TUMORS

A. Ewing's Sarcoma (Endothelioma)
    1. Incidence
        Can occur in children under 10 years, but peak incidence occurs during second decade
    2. Pathology
        a. Arises from metaphysis or diaphysis
        b. Primarily involves femur, pelvis, humerus, tibia, or rib cage
        c. Tumor composed of small round cells similar to those found in neuroblastoma, lymphoma, embryonal rhabdosarcoma
        d. Metastasizes to lungs, bone, bone marrow, central nervous system, abdominal viscera (rare)
    3. Manifestations
        a. Pain, swelling of involved area most common presenting symptoms
        b. Fever and elevated sedimentation rate occur occasionally
        c. Diffuse osteolytic lesion with indefinite borders and periosteal elevation seen on roentgenograms
    4. Diagnosis
        a. Clinical signs and symptoms
        b. Roentgenographic findings
        c. Biopsy
        d. Because histology is not definitive, additional tests should be made to rule out lymphoma, neuroblastoma, embryonal rhabdosarcoma
            1. Bone scan
            2. Serum tests including BUN, Ca, P, alkaline phosphatase levels
            3. Chest tomography
            4. Intravenous pyelogram
            5. Urine (24-hour) for HVA and VMA
            6. Bone marrow aspirate and biopsy
            7. Lumbar puncture
    5. Prognosis
        Extremely poor
    6. Treatment
        a. Radiotherapy
        b. Chemotherapy
        c. Surgery usually not indicated because multiple areas are involved before diagnosis is made

B. Osteogenic sarcoma
1. Incidence
   a. Most common malignant bone tumor of children and adolescents
   b. Slightly more common in males
2. Pathology
   a. Affects growing end of fastest growing bones
   b. Predominantly involves adolescents
   c. Distal femur, proximal tibia, proximal humerus most commonly involved
   d. Metastatic spread to lungs, bone
3. Manifestations
   a. Pain, swelling, soft tissue mass
   b. Usually history of preceding trauma
   c. Osteolytic and sclerotic areas evident on roentgenogram
   d. Serum alkaline phosphatase frequently elevated
4. Diagnosis
   a. Clinical signs and symptoms
   b. Roentgenographic findings
   c. Biopsy
   d. Metastatic evaluation
      1. Chest film
      2. Bone scan
5. Prognosis
   Very poor, tumor is radioresistant
6. Treatment
   a. Surgery
      Amputation previously required but now limb salvage is possible using cadaver bone transplant to replace excised bone
   b. Chemotherapy

BIBLIOGRAPHY

Deelgy TJ: Modern Radiotherapy and Oncology. Malignant Diseases in Children. London, Butterworth, 1974

Evans AE, D'Angio GJ, Koop CE: Diagnosis and treatment of neuroblastoma. Pediatr Clin North Am 23:161–170, 1976

Jenkin RDT: The treatment of Wilm's tumor. Pediatr Clin North Am 23:147–160, 1976

Miller DR et al: Smith's Blood Diseases of Infancy and Childhood. Saint Louis, Mosby, 1978

Pinkel D: Treatment of acute leukemia. Pediatr Clin North Am 23:117–130, 1976

Rosen G: Management of malignant bone tumors in children and adolescents. Pediatr Clin North Am 23:183–214, 1976

Shurin SB: Infectious mononucleosis. Pediatr Clin North Am 26:315–326, 1979

Wintrobe WM et al: Clinical Hematology. Philadelphia, Lea & Febiger, 1974

10

Pediatric Neurology

SPINA BIFIDA, MENINGOCELE, MENINGOMYELOCELE (Figs. 73, 74)

A. Definitions
1. *Spina bifida occulta:* Failure of bony spine to close
2. *Meningocele:* Associated defect of meninges with protrusion of saclike mass of meninges covered by skin
3. *Meningomyelocele:* Extreme form of spina bifida with protrusion of mass containing neural tissue in addition to meninges

B. Etiology
1. Causes unknown but occur in early fetal life
2. May be familial
3. Hereditary factors may play an important role

C. Clinical and Laboratory Features
1. *Spina bifida occulta* as an isolated lesion is asymptomatic
2. Uncomplicated *meningocele* is also usually asymptomatic
3. *Meningomyelocele* causes neurologic symptoms
4. Dimple or localized hairy area sometimes overlies *spina bifida occulta.* Lipomatous tissue or bony defect may sometimes be palpated

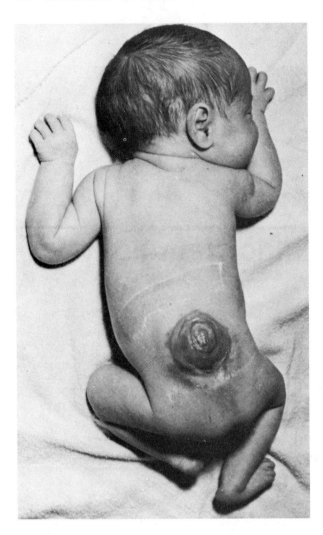

Fig. 73. Lumbar meningomyelocele in a 3-day-old infant. There is moderate weakness of the proximal muscle groups and more extensive weakness of the distal musculature in the lower extremities. The lesion was flat at birth but began to elevate in the next 2 days. (*Bell WE: In Schaffer AJ, Avery ME (eds): Diseases of the Newborn, p 754. Philadelphia, W. B. Saunders, 1977*)

    5. Hydrocephalus may be associated

    6. If cauda equina is involved, may have motor weakness and atrophy, bladder dysfunction, sensory loss, and absent reflexes in lower extremities. If spinal cord is involved, neurologic deficit corresponds to level of lesion

    7. Vertebral defects demonstrable on roentgenogram

D. Treatment

    1. *Spina bifida occulta* requires no treatment

    2. Simple *meningocele* is correctable surgically

    3. Meticulous care of skin essential for *meningomyelocele*. Indications for surgical correction somewhat controversial. Early surgery if paralysis and sphincter disorder are only partial and if no hydrocephalus is associated. Many centers do

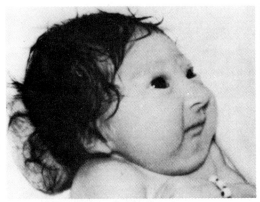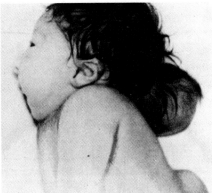

Fig. 74. Occipital meningoencephalocele. The sloping forehead and small head circumference are evident, although progressive ventricular enlargement often subsequently occurs in such children. (*Bell WE: In Schaffer AJ, Avery ME (eds): Diseases of the Newborn, p 736. Philadelphia, W. B. Saunders, 1977*)

not advocate surgery if paralysis of lower extremities is complete or if progressive hydrocephalus is present. However, some surgeons recommend excision of meningomyelocele despite neurologic status in order to improve nursing care

E. Prognosis
  1. Good with simple *meningocele* if closed surgically
  2. Majority of patients with untreated *meningomyelocele* (more than 90%) do not survive first year. Cause of death is infection

HYDROCEPHALUS (Fig. 75)

A. Definition
   Enlargement of ventricles with progressive cranial distention
B. Etiology
  1. Contributing factors include partial obstruction of cerebrospinal fluid flow within ventricular channels (particularly at foramen of Monro, third ventricle, aqueduct of Sylvius, foramen of Luschka, foramen of Magendie) or absorptive failure of cerebrospinal fluid (communicating hydrocephalus)
  2. Specific etiologic agents include arachnoidal fibrosis (following meningitis inflammatory reactions, subarachnoid hemorrhage), Arnold-Chiari malformation,* atresia of foramen of Magendie, anomalies of aqueduct of Sylvius, obstruction of pathways by neoplasms or aneurysms, some cases of achondrodysplasia
C. Clinical Features
  1. *In acute cases:* Nausea, vomiting, headache, lethargy, drowsiness, confusion
  2. *In chronic cases:* Progressive enlargement of head, which may become mas-

* See Glossary

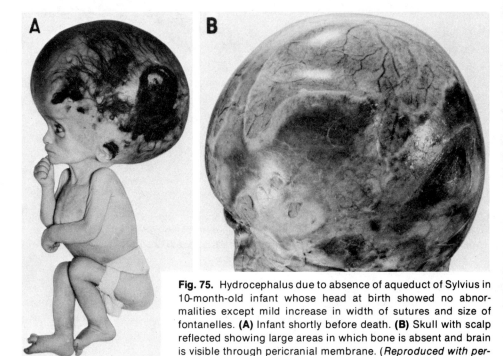

Fig. 75. Hydrocephalus due to absence of aqueduct of Sylvius in 10-month-old infant whose head at birth showed no abnormalities except mild increase in width of sutures and size of fontanelles. **(A)** Infant shortly before death. **(B)** Skull with scalp reflected showing large areas in which bone is absent and brain is visible through pericranial membrane. (*Reproduced with permission from Potter EL, Craig JM: Pathology of the Fetus and the Infant, 3rd edition. Copyright © 1975 by Year Book Medical Publishers, Inc., Chicago*)

sively enlarged. Mental deficiency and neurologic abnormalities may or may not be present. In severe cases, neurologic deficits may be severe

D. Diagnosis
 1. Rapidly enlarging head size
 2. Transillumination shows a halo extending more than 3 cm from rim of light source
 3. Roentgenogram may show honeycomb appearance of skull with multiple areas of translucency (craniolacunae)
 4. Roentgenogram of spine may show spina bifida occulta or abnormalities of cervical vertebrae
 5. CT scan of skull shows dilated ventricles

E. Treatment
 1. Treatment of choice for communicating hydrocephalus and for infantile noncommunicating hydrocephalus is shunting of cerebrospinal fluid to an extracranial compartment (superior vena cava or peritoneal cavity, latter generally preferred)
 2. Although some cases may arrest spontaneously, needless procrastination may result in later compromise of cognitive function and of motor coordination

F. Prognosis
   1. Mortality is 50% if untreated
   2. Mental retardation, impaired intellectual function in high proportion of cases
   3. Major physical handicaps common
   4. Neurologic defects include ataxia, spastic diplegia, compromised fine motor coordination, perceptual defects

MENTAL RETARDATION (MENTAL DEFICIENCY)

A. Definition
   1. Impairment of intellectual development, which impedes independent social adjustment at maturity
   2. May be congenital or acquired
   3. May be associated with a long list of disorders, or no underlying defect may be apparent
B. Incidence
   In about 3% of population (does not include persons who function at retarded level because of emotional or sociocultural factors but have normal intellectual potential)
C. Classification
   1. General classification
      a. Prenatal (includes genetic)
      b. Perinatal
      c. Postnatal
   2. Classification by intelligence level
      a. *Mild retardation:* IQ 55–69 (in 90%)
      b. *Moderate retardation:* IQ 40–54 (in 6%)
      c. *Severe retardation:* IQ 25–39
      d. *Profound retardation:* IQ less than 25
D. Significance of Classification
   1. *Mild* and some *moderate* cases are "educable"
   2. Some *moderate* and many *severe* cases are "trainable"
   3. Some *severe* and *profound* cases are considered "custodial"
E. Etiology
   1. Prenatal causes include genetic factors (*i.e.,* Down's syndrome and other trisomies), environmental factors affecting fetus (*i.e.,* radiation, maternal disease)
   2. Perinatal causes include anoxia, trauma, hyperbilirubinemia, infection
   3. Postnatal causes include trauma, infection, dehydration, poisonings, severe malnutrition, and others
F. Evaluation
   1. Early evaluation is important because it may uncover potentially correctable biochemical defect or provide opportunity for establishing optimal environment
   2. Best evaluated by a team representing various specialties such as pediatrics, neurology, psychiatry, psychology, social service, nursing. Other specialists (*i.e.,*

audiologists, speech therapists, ophthalmologists, physical therapists, orthopedists) may be needed

3. Management should be coordinated by a single individual (usually family physician, pediatrician, or pediatric neurologist)
4. Evaluation includes thorough history, observation of behavior, physical examination including neurologic evaluation, psychologic testing, evaluation of both vision and hearing. In selected cases, laboratory tests for inborn errors of metabolism (*i.e.*, galactosemia, phenylketonuria), and syphilis, skull roentgenograms, electroencephalogram, blood sugar, pneumoencephalography, cerebral angiography, chromosome studies, thyroid hormone levels (in suspected hypothyroidism), urinary uric acid levels (Lesch-Nyhan syndrome*). Laboratory tests selected depend on disorders suggested by clinical evaluation
5. Must be differentiated from various learning disabilities, from poor performance resulting from hearing or visual defects, emotional problems, sociocultural deprivation

G. Treatment
1. Specific therapy if underlying condition treatable
2. Most are not amenable to specific therapy
3. Counseling and guidance regarding education, training, and, in selected cases, placement away from home

CEREBRAL PALSY

A. Definition
1. A broad term including variety of syndromes affecting brain from birth or early life, manifest by impaired motor function (may also include learning disabilities, mental retardation, seizures)
2. *Not a specific* medical diagnosis
B. Etiology
1. Prenatal factors include a variety of genetic and acquired conditions that result in damage to fetal nervous system
2. Perinatal factors include asphyxia, cerebral hemorrhage, kernicterus
3. Postnatal factors include meningitis, encephalitis, marasmus, dehydration
C. Clinical Manifestations
1. Spastic cerebral palsy characterized by increased muscle tone, exaggerated deep tendon reflexes, extensor plantar response (positive Babinski sign), tendency to contractures
   a. *Hemiplegia:* Involvement of both extremities on same side
   b. *Quadraplegia:* Involvement of all four extremities
   c. *Diplegia:* Involvement of both lower extremities with lesser involvement of upper extremities
   d. *Paraplegia:* Involvement of both lower extremities only

* See Glossary

e. *Monoplegia:* Involvement of one extremity (rare)

f. *Triplegia:* Involvement of three extremities (rare)

2. *Dyskinetic cerebral palsy* characterized by purposeless uncontrolled slow wormlike or writhing movements while awake, usually involving face, neck, extremities, trunk (*athetosis*). If a jerky component is present, disorder is referred to as *choreoathetosis*

Usually related to lesions in basal ganglia (*i.e.,* kernicterus)

3. *Ataxic cerebral palsy* characterized by nonprogressive ataxia from early childhood

4. *Mixed forms of cerebral palsy* consist of two or more of the foregoing

5. Associated manifestations

a. Mental retardation (25–75%)

b. Seizure disorders

c. Speech disorders

d. Visual handicaps (strabismus, visual field defects, refractive errors)

e. Deafness and athetosis due to kernicterus

D. Diagnosis

Clinical manifestations

E. Treatment

1. Physical therapy

2. Surgical correction of contractures

3. Braces (contraindicated in athetosis)

4. Medication generally not successful in reducing spasticity, although diazepam (Valium) may be helpful in cases with strong emotional overlay. Dantrolene sodium (Dantrium) may produce some relaxation of skeletal muscles *used for malignant Neuroleptic Syn*

5. Anticonvulsants for seizures

6. Treatment of associated disorders

7. Family guidance and counseling

MIGRAINE AND MIGRAINE VARIANTS

A. General Considerations

1. A common disorder

2. Symptoms appear before 10 years of age in most patients

B. Definition

A disorder characterized by recurrent attacks of headache (frequently unilateral and varied in intensity, duration, and frequency), often associated with anorexia, nausea, vomiting, sensory and motor disturbances, and positive family history

C. Manifestations

1. *Classic form:* Sharply defined headache associated with prodrome of visual or other sensory or motor disturbances

2. *Common form:* No striking prodrome, and headaches less likely to be unilateral

3. *Cluster form:* Unilateral, closely recurrent headaches usually associated with ipsilateral nasal or lacrimal discharge

4. *Hemiplegic or ophthalmoplegic form:* Sensory and motor phenomena accompany headache and persist after headache subsides
5. Is recurrent in nature and accompanied by any three of the following symptoms: unilateral headache, abdominal pain, nausea or vomiting, pulsatile type of pain, relief after period of sleep, aura (visual, sensory, or motor). Also, may have family history of migraine
6. Associations sometimes include vertigo, motion sickness, dizziness, associated enuresis, nightmares, somnambulism*

D. Diagnosis
   1. Must exclude epilepsy, structural brain disease, tension headaches, headaches due to psychiatric disease, sinus headaches
   2. Clinical manifestations with positive family history and absence of seizures strongly favor diagnosis of migraine

E. Treatment and Prognosis
   1. High incidence of spontaneous improvement and total remission
   2. Analeptic drugs used prophylactically
   3. Salicylates or ergot drugs for acute attack
   4. Brief period of bed rest

SEIZURES

A. Acute Seizures
   1. Due to variety of disorders including cerebral hemorrhage, cerebral infections, toxic agents, anoxia, metabolic disorders, brain tumors, roseola infantum, shigellosis, febrile illnesses
   2. Febrile Seizures
      a. *Simple* seizures
         1. Generalized motor convulsions occurring shortly after the onset of an acute febrile disease (especially roseola infantum and shigella infection)
         2. Cause is unknown but probably is related to *rate of rise* of rather than to the height of temperature
         3. Age incidence is 6 months to 6 years
         4. Are of short duration and benign in nature
      b. *Complex* febrile seizures
         1. Include generalized convulsions greater than 15 minutes in duration, focal convulsions or cluster convulsions
         2. A greater proportion of these patients eventually develop idiopathic epilepsy or other evidence of neurologic disease
      c. Immediate treatment
         1. Sedation (phenobarbital, diazepam)
         2. Tepid sponges to reduce fever
         3. Antipyretics when conscious

* See Glossary

4. Some believe spinal fluid analysis should be routinely performed in *all* cases to exclude central nervous system infection (controversial)

d. Subsequent treatment

1. Complex seizures require complete neurologic examination. Also, an electroencephalogram should be obtained not less than 10 days after the episode. With prolonged seizures, metabolic evaluation is indicated

2. Some believe that daily prophylactic administration of phenobarbital is indicated and should be continued until patient is 6 years of age (controversial issue). However, most authorities do not believe that phenobarbital prophylaxis is justified unless seizures are recurrent (two or more illnesses) or unless there are other factors that place the patient in a high-risk category (*i.e.*, family history of epilepsy, neurologic abnormalities prior to the episode, abnormal electroencephalogram). Intermittent prophylaxis (with onset of febrile illness only) is not effective

B. Epilepsy

1. Definition

Chronic recurrent seizures considered *idiopathic* if no associated cause or *organic* if associated with other disorders

2. Types

a. *Grand mal seizures* (*major motor seizures*): Characterized by generalized tonic or clonic muscular contractions preceded by aura and followed by period of drowsiness (postictal state)

b. *Petit mal seizures:* Characterized by transient loss of consciousness (absence) of less than 30 seconds duration; rarely associated with falling; varying in frequency from occasional to several hundred a day

c. *Psychomotor seizures:* Characterized by a period of altered behavior that patient does not remember

d. *Focal seizures:* Localized motor or sensory symptoms

e. *Minor motor seizures:* Include akinetic seizures, myoclonic seizures, atypical petit mal, infantile spasms (hypsarrhythmia)

1. *Akinetic seizures:* Characterized by momentary loss of muscle tone. When loss of tone is partial, head and neck fall forward ("salaam seizure"). When loss of tone is generalized, child suddenly falls to ground. May occur several times during the day, but spontaneous remissions for days or weeks not uncommon

2. *Myoclonic seizures:* Characterized by single or repetitive contractures of a muscle or group of muscles

3. *Atypical petit mal seizures:* Characterized by absences but differs from true petit mal in that episodes occur in cycles and disappear for as long as several days at a time

4. *Infantile spasms:* Associated with many disorders including Sturge-Weber syndrome,* tuberous sclerosis, pyridoxine deficiency, phenylketonuria, hypoglycemia, hypocalcemia, lead encephalopathy. Onset

* See Glossary

1–13 months of age. Episodes consist of sudden flexing of head and of flexion or extension of arms and legs occurring in series of 8–10 and sometimes recurring over 100 times a day. Usually cease spontaneously at 3–4 years of age, but 75–90% become mentally retarded. ACTH may suppress seizures but response is usually temporary

3. Diagnosis
   a. Clinical manifestations
   b. Electroencephalogram
   c. Exclude organic causes
4. Treatment
   a. *Major motor seizures:* phenytoin (Dilantin), primidone (Mysoline), carbamazepine (Tegretol), mephenytoin (Mesantoin), mephobarbital (Mebaral)
   b. *Petit mal seizures:* ethosuximide (Zarontin), clonazepam (Clonopin), trimethadione (Tridione), paramethadione (Paradione), methsuximide (Celontin), quinacrine hydrochloride (Atabrine)
   c. *Psychomotor seizures:* phenytoin (Dilantin), carbamazepine (Tegretol), primidone (Mysoline), phenobarbital, mephobarbital (Mebaral), phenacemide (Phenurone)
   d. *Minor motor seizures:* clonazepam (Clonopin), diazepam (Valium), primidone (Mysoline), ketogenic diet
   e. *Focal seizures:* phenytoin (Dilantin), primidone (Mysoline), phenobarbital
   f. *Infantile spasms:* nitrazepam (Mogadon), corticotropin (ACTH)

BRAIN TUMORS

A. General Considerations
   1. Most common neoplasms in children next to leukemia
   2. Occur at any age but mostly 5–10 years
   3. Cerebellar tumors most common
B. Manifestations
   Increased intracranial pressure: Hydrocephalus, headache, vomiting (unaccompanied by nausea), hypertension, bradycardia, papilledema, drowsiness, sixth nerve palsy with blurring of vision or diploplia, loss of visual acuity due to optic nerve damage
C. Classification
   1. *Cerebellar astrocytoma:* If completely resectable, cure rate is 90%
   2. *Medulloblastoma:* A midline cerebellar tumor. Prognosis grave
   3. *Ependymoma:* Arises from ependymal lining of floor of fourth ventricle. Prognosis grave
   4. *Glioma of brain stem:* Characterized by bilateral cranial nerve palsies, pyramidal tract signs (hyperreflexia and Babinski sign), ataxia, usually with no evidence of increased intracranial pressure. Prognosis grave
   5. *Craniopharyngioma:* Sellar or suprasellar in location and associated with

hypothalamic and pituitary dysfunction. Symptoms include growth failure, progressive visual loss, increased intracranial pressure, diabetes insipidus, delayed puberty. Cure by surgical excision possible but difficult

D. Diagnosis
   1. Clinical manifestations
   2. Roentgenogram of skull shows spreading of sutures, digital markings. With craniopharyngioma, suprasellar calcification (80%) and enlarged sella turcica
   3. Pneumoencephalography
   4. Cerebral angiography
   5. Radionuclide brain scan
   6. CT scan

E. Treatment
   1. Surgical excision if possible
   2. Radiation for medulloblastoma, cytoxic drugs in selected cases

HEAD INJURY

A. Minor Head Trauma
   1. If no loss of consciousness, hospitalization not indicated
   2. Dizziness, nausea, vomiting, headache commonly occur
   3. Marked or progressive lethargy requires reevaluation

B. Concussion
   1. Head injury followed by loss of consciousness and amnesia of events surrounding injury
   2. Severity proportional to duration of unconsciousness and extent of amnesia
   3. Due to jarring of brain
   4. Roentgenograms are necessary to exclude fracture
   5. Observe at home if period of unconsciousness is less than 5 minutes and if child regains normal state of alertness

C. Skull Fracture
   1. Must observe for intracranial hemorrhage
   2. Many prefer to hospitalize child for 24 hours of observation
   3. Significantly depressed fractures require surgical elevation
   4. Basal skull fractures require hospitalization and may be complicated by meningitis
   5. Skull fracture in infants may be complicated by leptomeningeal cyst, which causes defect in skull to enlarge (spreading fracture). Surgical resection may be required

D. Severe Head Injury
   1. Prolonged period of unconsciousness with contusion or laceration of brain tissue
   2. May be complicated by intracranial hemorrhage and edema
   3. Neuroradiologic studies and surgical intervention may be indicated
   4. Hospitalization essential, prognosis guarded

E. Subdural Hematoma
1. Bleeding into subdural space. Almost always associated with hemorrhage of underlying brain
2. May become chronic with signs of increasing intracranial pressure
3. Diagnosis best established by CT scan
4. If symptomatic, repeated subdural taps or surgical drainage required

ATAXIAS

A. Definition

Muscular incoordination
B. Common Causes in Children
1. Phenytoin (Dilantin) toxicity is most common cause
2. Brain tumors
3. Acute cerebellar ataxia (transient disorder associated with infectious disease)
4. Ataxia-Telangectasia (Fig. 76)
a. Progressive cerebellar degeneration associated with telangectasia of conjunctiva and skin and with immunologic dysfunction
b. Autosomal recessive
c. Prone to develop malignancy
d. Manifestations usually begin in infancy with progressive dysarthria,* nystagmus, intention tremor, choreoathetosis. Tendon reflexes diminished or absent
e. Slow progressive course with death in adolescence
5. Friedreich's Ataxia
a. Autosomal recessive transmission
b. Onset in late childhood or adolescence
c. Manifestations include progressive gait disturbance, pes cavus (high arched foot), scoliosis, gait ataxia, dysarthria, intention tremor, nystagmus, cardiac failure, peripheral neuropathy, muscle weakness and atrophy, reduced or absent tendon reflexes
d. Positive Babinski sign plus absent ankle jerks is almost pathognomonic
e. No effective treatment

FAMILIAL DYSAUTONOMIA (RILEY-DAY SYNDROME)

A. General Considerations
1. Disturbance in autonomic and peripheral sensory functions
2. Autosomal recessive transmission
3. In Ashkenazi Jews

* See Glossary

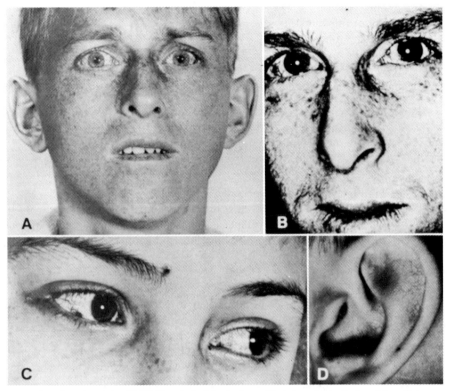

Fig. 76. Ataxia-telangiectasia. **(A,B)** The dull, thin facies with telangiectasia involving the eyes and bridge of the nose. **(C,D)** Close-ups of telangiectasia of the eyes and ear. (*Miller SJH, Gooddy W: Brain 87:581, 1964*)

B. Manifestations
1. Fungiform papillae of tongue reduced or absent
2. Poor swallowing, excessive bronchial secretions, repeated aspiration with recurrent pneumonia
3. Excessive salivation, excessive sweating, absence of tear formation, labile hypertension and orthostatic hypotension, periodic fevers, blotchy skin (autonomic disturbances)
4. Absence of taste sensation, diminished sense of pain, reduced or absent corneal reflex (peripheral sensory dysfunction)
5. Dysarthria, clumsiness, emotional lability
C. Diagnosis
1. Clinical manifestations
2. Methacholine chloride (Mecholyl) test (pupil responds to methacholine chloride instillation by constriction); no response in normal people
3. Histamine test (no flare or pain response to intradermal injection of histamine)

D. Treatment
   1. Control of infections
   2. Family support
E. Prognosis
   1. Poor
   2. Most succumb from chronic pulmonary failure before reaching adult life

WILSON'S DISEASE (HEPATOLENTICULAR DEGENERATION)

A. General Considerations
   1. Transmitted as autosomal recessive
   2. Disorder of copper metabolism resulting in injury to basal ganglia and liver
   3. Defect in synthesis of ceruloplasmin (a copper-carrying protein) is basis of disorder. Decreased protein binding of serum copper leads to accumulation of copper in tissues
B. Manifestations
   1. Subacute or chronic hepatic failure in early childhood
   2. Neurologic abnormalities usually occur in later childhood or adolescence
   3. Flapping tremor of shoulders and wrists characteristic ("wing-beating" tremor)
   4. Dysarthria, choreoathetoid movements, rigidity, drooling
   5. Rarely spasticity, hermiparesis, positive Babinski sign
   6. May have mental changes with no other neurologic signs
   7. May have emotional lability, school failure, frank psychosis
   8. Kayser-Fleisher ring (greenish yellow rim of cornea resulting from copper-deposit). Usually visible but may require slit-lamp examination
C. Diagnosis
   1. Low serum ceruloplasmin
   2. High urine copper values that increase after administration of penicillamine
   3. Neurologic manifestations plus evidence of liver disease
D. Prognosis
   Usually fatal within five years of onset
E. Treatment
   Penicillamine therapy plus diet low in copper

LEARNING DISORDERS (CEREBRAL DYSFUNCTION)

A. General Considerations
   1. Includes children with learning or behavior disorders who are not mentally deficient and who have no recognizable neurologic defects
   2. Synonym is "minimal cerebral dysfunction syndrome"

B. Manifestations
   1. Unpredictable variations of behavior, short attention span, hyperactivity, impulsiveness, irritability, perceptual and conceptual difficulties, poor motor coordination, sleep disorders, easy frustration
   2. School-age child shows reading disability, poor organization, difficulty in following instructions, in learning, and in memory . . . all leading to poor performance in school
C. Diagnosis
   1. Clinical manifestations
   2. Must exclude hearing and visual defects, mental deficiency, neurologic disease
D. Treatment
   1. Consultation with teachers and parents
   2. Special classes available in some schools
   3. Drug therapy includes dextroamphetamine sulfate (Dexedrine), methylphenidate hydrochloride (Ritalin), chlorpromazine hydrochloride (Thorazine), thioridazine hydrochloride (Mellaril), diphenhydramine hydrochloride (Benadryl)
E. Prognosis
   With proper guidance, most children adjust during adolescence

BIBLIOGRAPHY

Farmer TW: Pediatric Neurology. Hagerstown, Harper & Row, 1975

Menkes JH: Textbook of Child Neurology. Philadelphia, Lea & Febiger, 1974

Menkes JH: Diagnosis and treatment of minor motor seizures. Pediatr Clin North Am 23:435–442, 1976

Prensky AL: Migraine and migrainous variants in pediatric patients. Pediatr Clin North Am 23:461–469, 1976

Rudolph AM, Barnett HL, Einhorn AH: Pediatrics. New York, Appleton-Century-Crofts, 1977

11

Pediatric Endocrinology

ADRENOGENITAL SYNDROME
(CONGENITAL ADRENAL HYPERPLASIA) (Figs. 77, 78)

A. General Considerations
1. Definition
   Failure to synthesize cortisol secondary to enzyme deficiency, which results in cortical hyperfunction and ambiguous genitalia, salt-losing crises, virilization, rarely hypertension
2. Genitalia
   a. *Female:* With some enzyme deficiencies, excessive androgens are produced. They cause fusion of vaginal outlet and enlarged clitoris (ambiguous genitalia) at birth
   b. *Male:* Excessive androgens cause enlarged phallus at birth with subsequent virilization if untreated
3. Autosomal recessive transmission
4. Occurs in 1 of about 100,000 live births
B. 21-Hydroxylase Deficiency
1. Most common form (about 90%)

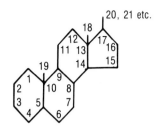

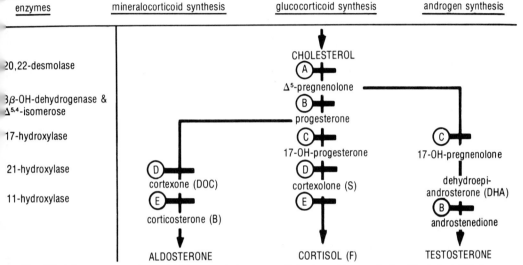

enzymes	mineralocorticoid synthesis	glucocorticoid synthesis	androgen synthesis
		CHOLESTEROL	
20,22-desmolase		(A)	
		Δ^5-pregnenolone	
3β-OH-dehydrogenase & $\Delta^{5,4}$-isomerose		(B)	
		progesterone	
17-hydroxylase		(C)	(C)
		17-OH-progesterone	17-OH-pregnenolone
21-hydroxylase	(D)	(D)	
	cortexone (DOC)	cortexolone (S)	dehydroepi-androsterone (DHA)
11-hydroxylase	(E)	(E)	(B)
	corticosterone (B)		androstenedione
	ALDOSTERONE	CORTISOL (F)	TESTOSTERONE

Fig. 77. Inborn errors of steroid biogenesis in congenital adrenal hyperplasia. (*Zurbrügg RP: In Gardner LI (ed): Endocrine and Genetic Diseases of Childhood and Adolescence, p 478. Philadelphia, W. B. Saunders, 1975*)

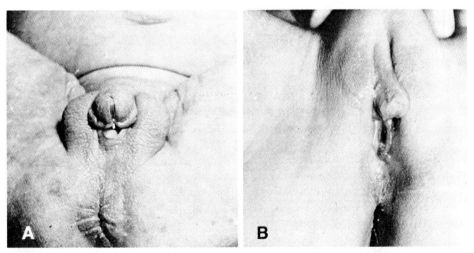

Fig. 78. Genitalia of girl with congenital adrenal hyperplasia. **(A)** External genitalia, age 1 month. Note clitoral enlargement. **(B)** External genitalia, age 3 years, 8 months, after steroid treatment and opening of only the urogenital sinus. The clitoris eventually became much less prominent; therefore, no surgical removal was required. (*Zurbrügg RP: In Gardner LI (ed): Endocrine and Genetic Diseases of Childhood and Adolescence p 494. Philadelphia, W. B. Saunders, 1975*)

2. Most important feature is *virilization*
3. If untreated, patient develops accelerated growth and development, premature pubic and axillary hair, acne, growth of phallus
4. Diagnosis by clinical signs and symptoms, serum 17-hydroxyprogesterone (markedly elevated)
5. Salt-losing crisis
   a. Due to aldosterone deficiency
   b. Occurs in about one-half of these patients
   c. Usually occurs 10–12 days after birth
   d. Symptoms include poor feeding, vomiting
   e. Serum sodium is abnormally low whereas serum potassium, urea nitrogen, and creatinine are elevated
   f. Dehydration occurs rapidly
6. Treatment (salt-losing type)
   a. Regular physical examinations
   b. Intravenous fluids
   c. Mineralocorticoid (desoxycorticosterone acetate, DOCA)
   d. Cortisol
   e. Discontinuance of drug therapy in salt losers can cause acute adrenal insufficiency

C. 11-Hydroxylase Deficiency
   1. About 5% of all cases
   2. Deficiency of cortisol with excess of mineralocorticoid
   3. No salt-losing crisis
   4. Develop salt retention and occasionally hypertension
   5. Treat with cortisone
D. 3 Beta-Dehydrogenase Deficiency
   1. Rare
   2. Can have salt loss
E. 17-Hydroxylase Deficiency
   Rare

DIABETES MELLITUS (JUVENILE DIABETES MELLITUS, INSULIN-DEPENDENT DIABETES MELLITUS)

A. Definition
   Subnormal or absent levels of insulin secondary to defective pancreatic activity resulting in hyperglycemia, polyuria, polydipsia, polyphagia
B. Incidence and Associations
   1. Most common endocrine-metabolic disease in pediatrics
   2. No sex predominance
   3. High incidence of diabetes following mumps epidemics

C. Clinical Manifestations
   1. Presents with polyuria, polydipsia, polyphagia, weight loss
   2. Lethargy, weakness common
   3. Insidious onset
   4. Occasionally presents with ketoacidosis (about 10–20%)
      a. *Symptoms:* Air hunger, Kussmaul respirations* (seen with acidosis), obtundation* or coma, vomiting, dehydration
      b. Ketonemia, hyperglycemia, glycosuria, ketonuria
   5. Abnormal glucose tolerance test
D. Diagnosis
   1. Clinical signs and symptoms
   2. Urinalysis
   3. Blood sugar
   4. Glucose tolerance test
E. Complications
   1. Ketoacidosis
      a. Hyperglycemia
      b. Ketonemia
      c. Acidosis
      d. Glycosuria, ketonuria
      e. Precipitated by trauma, infection, vomiting, psychologic disturbances
      f. Dehydration major concern
   2. Nonketotic hyperosmolar coma
      a. Rare in children
      b. Glucose greater than 500 mg per dl
      c. Elevated serum osmolality
   3. Hypoglycemia
      a. *Signs and symptoms:* Trembling, shaking, sweating, apprehension, tachycardia, hunger, drowsiness, mental confusion, seizure, coma
      b. Caused by inadequate coloric intake or excessive insulin dosage
      c. Treat by giving food with sugar (candy) to patient
   4. Posthypoglycemic hyperglycemia (Somogyi effect)
      a. Due to excessive insulin
      b. Patient has hyperglycemia, ketosis, ketonuria following mildly symptomatic hypoglycemia
      c. Unstable diabetes despite increasing doses of insulin suggestive of this phenomenon. Requires reduction of insulin dosage
   5. Retinopathy
      a. Develop microaneurysms, exudates, hemorrhages, invasion of blood vessels and fibrous tissue into vitreous (retinitis proliferans)
      b. Slowly progressive disease
      c. Can occur in well-controlled diabetics

* See Glossary

  d. A leading cause of blindness
  e. Treatment by photocoagulation
6. Nephropathy
  a. Two types
    1. *Nodular glomerulosclerosis:* Glomerular disease characterized by nodular deposits of PAS positive material seen in mesangium. Can progress to complete glomerulosclerosis and uremia (Kimmelstiel-Wilson disease, extremely rare in childhood)
    2. *Tubular nephrosis:* Manifested by glycogen deposition in proximal tubules
  b. About 3% incidence
  c. First clinical sign is proteinuria
  d. Hypertension, increased BUN, edema can occur in varied degrees
  e. Not usually seen until mid to late teens
7. Neuropathy
  a. Manifested by decreased reflexes, paresis, decreased pain sensation in legs, increased sweating of feet, interosseous muscle atrophy
  b. Usually becomes evident 8–10 years after onset of disease
8. Infections
  a. Especially prone to develop urinary tract infections caused by bacteria or Candida albicans
  b. At risk for developing pyelonephritis (especially with papillary necrosis)
9. Cataracts
F. Treatment
  1. Diet
    a. No special diet, but nutritional requirements must be met
    b. 100 cal per kg per day for first 10 kg, 50 cal per kg for next 10 kg, 20 cal per kg from then on
    c. Caloric intake can be given as 2/10 each for breakfast and lunch, 3/10 for dinner, 1/10 each for midmorning, afternoon, and evening snacks
  2. Unrestricted exercise
  3. Insulin
  4. "Honeymoon" phase
    a. Progressive reduction of insulin requirement because of recurrent hypoglycemia
    b. Seen in at least 50% of children after initial presentation and stabilization
    c. Some patients maintain normal serum glucose levels without insulin treatment
    d. May last as long as 1–2 years
  5. Ketoacidosis
    a. Fluid and electrolyte therapy
    b. Require potassium (because correction of acidosis causes decrease in serum potassium)
    c. Bicarbonate usually not given unless pH less than 7.20
    d. Constant infusion of low dose of insulin

e. Ketone measurement
   1. Test only measures acetoacetate and acetone
   2. Ratio of betahydroxybutyrate to acetoacetate is about 3 : 1 but can be 8 : 1
   3. Correction of acidosis causes betahydroxybutyrate to dissociate and become acetoacetate
   4. Ketone measurement paradoxically rises during initial treatment
   5. Not a good indicator for evaluating effect of treatment
6. Nonketotic hyperosmolar coma
   a. Fluid and electrolyte therapy
   b. Insulin can cause rapid fall of glucose and osmolality, inducing cerebral edema, so should be given with extreme caution

DIABETES INSIPIDUS

A. Definition
   Disorder caused by lack of secretion or increased degradation of antidiuretic hormone (ADH)
B. Acquired Diabetes Insipidus
   1. Etiology
      a. Tumors most frequently implicated
      b. Can be caused by encephalitis, meningitis, head trauma
   2. Manifestations
      a. Usually abrupt onset polydipsia, polyuria, weakness, fatigue
      b. In cases caused by tumor, headaches, vomiting, symptoms associated with anterior pituitary deficiency may occur
      c. Skull films may show widening of sella, calcification (craniopharyngioma)
      d. Dilute urine with increased serum osmolality
   3. Diagnosis
      a. Clinical signs and symptoms
      b. Skull film
      c. Urinalysis
      d. Serum osmolality
   4. Complications
      Dehydration
   5. Treatment
      IM vasopressin tannate in oil
C. Congenital Diabetes Insipidus
   1. Nephrogenic diabetes insipidus*
      a. Manifestations
         1. Polydipsia, polyuria early after birth
         2. Constipation, unexplained fever, failure to gain weight

* Defect is in kidney, mechanism unknown

     b. Diagnosis
        1. As described previously but fails to respond to vasopressin
        2. Family history of disease
     c. Complications
        1. Dehydration
        2. Convulsions
        3. Mental retardation
        4. Hyperuricemia
     d. Treatment
        1. Low-salt diet
        2. Thiazide diuretics
        3. Spironolactone
  2. Familial diabetes insipidus due to vasopressin deficiency
     a. Etiology unknown
     b. Wide variability of symptoms
     c. Symptoms increase in severity with age
        Usually most severe in adolescence and adulthood
     d. Diagnosis as described previously
     e. Treatment with vasopressin

HYPOTHYROIDISM (Figs. 79, 80)

A. Congenital
  1. Etiology
     a. Aplasia or hypoplasia, ectopic gland, defective hormone, iodine deficiency, maternal radioactive iodine treatment, autoimmune thyroiditis, hypopituitarism
     b. Aplasia, hypoplasia, ectopic gland account for about 80% of cases
     c. One-third of all hypothyroidism is congenital
  2. Manifestations
     a. Usually normal looking at birth
     b. Prolonged gestation, macrosomia, constipation, poor feeding, prolonged jaundice
     c. Infrequently, puffy face, large fontanelles, large tongue
     d. Large goiters rarely present at birth
  3. Diagnosis
     a. Clinical signs and symptoms are not helpful early because irreversible brain damage may take place before symptoms are evident
     b. Low serum T_4 and elevated TSH
  4. Complications
     a. Mental retardation
     b. Delayed somatic growth, bone development, tooth eruption
     c. Ataxia, strabismus, spastic diplegia
  5. Treatment
     Thyroid hormone preparations

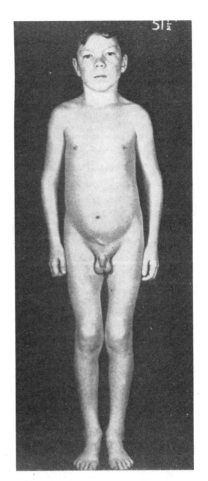

Fig. 79. Juvenile hypothyroidism in a boy, aged 17. Dwarfism and delayed sexual development are apparent. Trunk is longer than legs. Appearance is youthful. (*Ingbar SH, Woeber KA: In Williams RH (ed): Textbook of Endocrinology, p 199 Philadelphia, W. B. Saunders, 1974*)

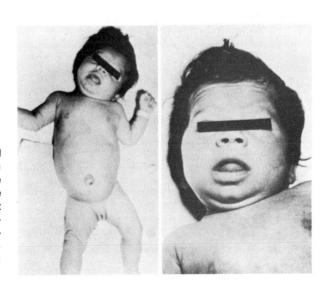

Fig. 80. Signs of congenital hypothyroidism are apparent in this 3½-month-old infant. Note the puffy facial features, large protruding tongue, protuberant abdomen, umbilical hernia, mottled skin, and hypotonic posture. (*LaFranchi SH: Hypothyroidism. Pediatr Clin North Am 26:33, 1979*)

B. Acquired
    1. Etiology
       a. Chronic lymphatic thyroiditis (Hashimoto's thyroiditis) most frequent cause
       b. Thyroidectomy, hypopituitarism, cystinosis, histiocytosis
    2. Manifestations
       a. Can be slow in onset
       b. Goiter with decreased growth rate most common presenting complaint
       c. Puffiness, lethargy, cold intolerance, bradycardia, obesity, myxedema,* delayed reflexes, precocious sex development
       d. Low serum T_4, normal or low serum T_3 resin uptake, elevated TSH
    3. Diagnosis
       a. Clinical signs and symptoms
       b. Serum T_4, T_3 resin uptake, TSH
       c. Antithyroglobulin antibodies (for thyroiditis)
    4. Treatment
       Thyroid hormone preparations

HYPERTHYROIDISM (GRAVE'S DISEASE)

A. Neonatal Grave's Disease
    1. Acquired from transplacental passage of thyroid-stimulating immunoglobulins [long-acting thyroid stimulator (LATS), LATS-protector (LATS-P)]
    2. Hyperthyroidism acquired in about 1% of infants of mothers with history of Grave's disease
    3. Infant can get disorder if mother euthyroid during pregnancy (especially if mother is treated by subtotal thyroidectomy)
    4. 1:1 male to female ratio
    5. Infants frequently premature with tachycardia and dyspnea
    6. Goiter and exophthalmos* not always present
    7. Accelerated bone development and premature closure of sutures frequently present
    8. Patient can develop congestive heart failure
    9. Diagnosis by history, signs, symptoms, elevated serum T_3 and T_4 levels
   10. Treatment
       a. Propranolol to alleviate cardiovascular stress
       b. Propylthiouracil
       c. Corticosteroids if disease is severe
   11. Disease disappears when thyroid-stimulating immunoglobulins are cleared from blood (usually occurs fairly rapidly)
B. Acquired Grave's Disease
    1. Most common cause of pediatric thyrotoxicosis
    2. Occurs more frequently in females

* See Glossary

3. Slow onset
4. Nervousness, increased sweating, heat intolerance, tremor, increased appetite, palpitations, goiter, exophthalmos, tachycardia usually present (Fig. 81)
5. Diagnosis by clinical signs and symptoms, elevated serum T_3, T_4, and low TSH levels
6. Treatment
   a. Prophylthiouracil
   b. Radioactive iodine
   c. Surgery

ADDISON'S DISEASE (HYPOADRENOCORTICISM)

General Considerations
1. Autoimmune disease most frequent cause
2. May be associated with Hashimoto's disease, hypoparathyroidism, diabetes mellitus, hypopituitarism, hypogonadism
3. Also may be associated with alopecia totalis,* vitiligo,* café au lait spots*
4. Progressive weakness and hyperpigmentation characteristic of the disease
5. Glucocorticoid insufficiency demonstrated by hypoglycemia, anorexia, muscular weakness
6. Dehydration, high urine sodium, hyponatremia, hyperkalemia, anemia, hypotension are result of aldosterone insufficiency
7. Diagnosis by signs, symptoms, serum electrolytes, urine electrolytes, ACTH plasma radioimmunoassay
8. Differentiation of primary (adrenal) and secondary (hypothalamic pituitary) adrenal insufficiency
   a. Metyrapone test
      1. Inhibits cortisol synthesis and causes accumulation of compound S
      2. Low serum compound S level after administration of metyrapone indicates hypofunction
   b. Serum cortisol measurement after administration of ACTH compound
      1. Low level indicates adrenal gland disorder
      2. Elevated level indicates pituitary or hypothalamic disorder
9. Treatment
   a. Glucocorticoids (corticosteroid)
   b. Mineralocorticoids (Florinef)

OVARIAN TUMORS

A. General Considerations
   1. These neoplasms are most frequent genital tumor of childhood

* See Glossary

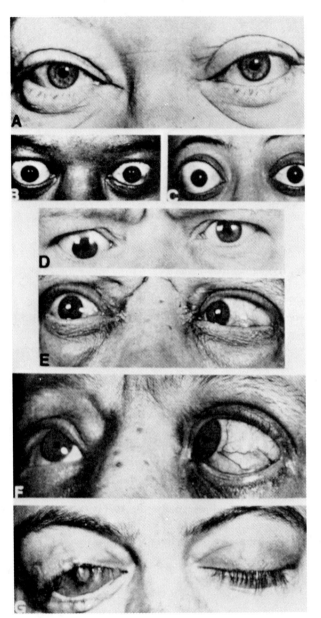

Fig. 81. Infiltrative ophthalmopathy in Grave's disease. **(A)** Palpebral edema. This patient's eyeballs protruded anteriorly 1 cm more than normal because of edema of the surrounding structures, but, there is no "pop-eye" appearance. **(B)** Widening of palpebral fissures; slight palpebral swelling. **(C)** Unequal degress of ophthalmopathy. **(D)** Unilateral lid retraction. **(E)** Palpebral swelling, presumably due to fat pads and edema; paralysis of right external rectus muscle. **(F)** Conjunctival injection and chemosis, together with ophthalmoplegia. **(G)** Failure to close lids on right due to marked exophthalmos, corneal scarring, and panophthalmitis; eye had to be enucleated. (*Ingbar SH, Woeber KA: In Williams RH (ed): Textbook of Endocrinology, p 172. Philadelphia, W. B. Saunders, 1974*)

2. Account for about 17% of all childhood neoplasms
3. Majority are benign
4. Types of neoplasms
    a. Functional cyst
        1. Variation of normal physiology
        2. Many present as asymptomatic mass and resolve in 1–2 months
        3. Sometimes menstrual irregularity and pain are presenting symptoms
        4. Complications include hemorrhage secondary to rupture, sexual precocity resulting from hormone secretion
    b. Teratoma-dermoid tumors
        1. Constitute about 30% of ovarian tumors
        2. Majority are benign
        3. High incidence of bilaterality (about 10–25%)
        4. Tumors are either cystic (dermoid) or solid (teratoma)
        5. Roentgenogram may show calcification (usually indicates benignancy)
B. Clinical Manifestations
    1. Tumor usually discovered fortuitously by mother or physician
    2. Chronic abdominal pain can be present
        Pain may mimic appendicitis or peritonitis
    3. Other symptoms include nausea, vomiting, urinary frequency or retention
C. Diagnosis
    1. Signs and symptoms
    2. Bimanual examination
    3. Ultrasound
D. Treatment
    1. Monthly examination to assess progress of mass
    2. If mass is large on initial presentation or if mass does not resolve after 3 months, then laparoscopy is indicated

TESTICULAR NEOPLASMS

A. General Considerations
    1. Most commonly seen in infants and adolescents
    2. Majority (about 60%) occur in patients younger than 2½ years
    3. Cryptorchidism associated with higher incidence of these tumors
B. Tumors of Infants and Children
    1. Majority (about 80%) are malignant
    2. Types
        a. Embryonal cell carcinoma
            1. Most common testicular tumor
            2. Usually presents in infancy
            3. Painless enlargement most common sign
            4. May present as hydrocele

   b. Sarcoma
      1. Second most frequent testicular neoplasm
      2. Patients present in early to mid childhood
      3. Presents as painless enlargement
      4. Can be confused with hydrocele
   c. Teratoma
      1. Seen in infancy and early childhood
      2. Presents as painless enlargement
      3. Usually benign
   d. Teratocarcinoma, choriocarcinoma, interstitial cell tumors rarely seen
3. Diagnosis by signs. Biopsy should be done if diagnosis in doubt
4. Treatment
   a. Surgery (orchiectomy, lymph node dissection)
   b. Chemotherapy and radiotherapy if lymph nodes are involved
C. Tumors of Adolescents
   1. Seminoma
      a. Originates from germinal cell
      b. Rare in childhood
      c. Cryptorchidism associated with higher incidence
      d. Usually presents as painless testicular mass
      e. Can present with symptoms from metastases (dyspnea, cough, hemoptysis, chest pain)
      f. Diagnosis by signs and symptoms
      g. Metastatic spread occurs to lymph nodes, lungs, liver, kidneys, pancreas, brain, bone
      h. Metastatic work-up includes lymphangiography, intravenous pyelogram, chest film, radionuclide studies of liver, bone
      i. Treatment includes surgery plus radiotherapy (especially effective) and chemotherapy
   2. Teratoma
      a. Occurs during first three decades
      b. Malignancy much more common in adolescents and adults than in infants and children
      c. Usually are cystic
      d. All three germ cell layers usually present
      e. Usually presents as painless testicular mass
      f. Diagnosis by signs and excisional biopsy
      g. Metastatic spread to lymph nodes, liver, lungs, bones
      h. Treatment consists of surgery, chemotherapy

SHORT STATURE

A. Definition
   No universal agreement, probably below two standard deviations; dwarfism below three standard deviations

B. Constitutional Short Stature
1. Majority of patients presenting with short stature have delayed puberty and will eventually reach normal adult height
2. Generally family history of delayed puberty
3. Physical examination reveals delayed secondary sexual development and growth curve below third percentile but parallel to normal
4. Roentgenogram of hand shows bone age less than chronological age
5. Arm-span-to-height and upper-body-to-lower-body ratios within normal limits
6. No treatment necessary

C. Growth Hormone Deficiency (Pituitary Dwarfism)
1. Occurs secondary to congenital defect, neoplasm, trauma, infection (*i.e.*, tuberculous meningitis), radiation therapy
2. Rarely familial
3. Patients are short and fail to grow at normal rate
4. Growth curve shows progressive deviation from normal
5. Normal body proportions
6. Obesity common
7. Congenital form usually presents with convulsions, cyanosis, shock (panhypopituitarism)
8. Diagnosis by signs and symptoms, bone age, roentgenograms, lack of serum growth hormone response to standardized stimuli
9. Treat with human growth hormone

D. Familial or Genetic (Primordial Dwarfism)
1. Patients are short for racial or ethnic background but not for family
2. Pubertal growth occurs at same time as general population
3. Short at birth
4. Growth well below third percentile but growth curve is parallel to normal
5. Bone age similar to chronological age
6. Serum growth hormone levels normal
7. No medical treatment helps
8. Psychosocial therapy may be beneficial

E. Idiopathic Intrauterine Growth Retardation
1. Underweight, short for gestational age with no associated anomalies
2. Sporadic incidence
3. Many patients reach normal adult height
4. Some never reach normal height
5. As neonate, may present with hypoglycemia
6. Growth curve parallel to normal
7. Bone age similar to chronological age
8. Diagnosis by signs and history, normal serum growth hormone
9. No treatment available
10. Psychosocial therapy may be beneficial

F. Developmental (Psychosocial)
1. Short stature associated with retardation of motor and personality development
2. Short stature may be due to undernutrition

3. Deviation from normal on growth curve
4. Delay in bone age
5. Treatment consists of psychosocial evaluation and therapy with possible foster home placement

OBESITY

A. Etiology and Pathogenesis
   1. Good predictor is rapid weight gain during first year of life
   2. Overwhelming majority of cases not organically based
   3. Hypothyroidism
      a. Seldom causes massive weight gain
      b. Patient plump, edematous, growth delay, delayed bone age, dry skin, constipation
      c. Serum T_4 for screening
   4. Hypercortisolism
      a. Most often caused by exogenous steroid therapy
      b. May be secondary to tumor, overproduction of ACTH (Cushing's syndrome)
      c. Usually presents with hypertension, thin dermal connective tissue, growth failure
      d. Dexamethasone suppression test for diagnosis
   5. Hypothalamic tumor, Prader-Willi syndrome,* Laurence-Moon-Biedl syndrome*
   6. Functional
      a. About 80% of obese adolescents become obese adults
      b. High caloric intake primary cause
      c. Decreased exercise and decreased food utilization also play significant role
      d. Diagnosis made by symptoms and signs
B. Complications
   1. More prone to developing furunculosis and acanthosis nigricans
   2. Slipped capital femoral epiphyses
   3. Implications of increased risk of hypertension, atherosclerosis, diabetes mellitus
C. Treatment
   1. Caloric restriction
   2. Psychosocial therapy
   3. Support

BIBLIOGRAPHY

LaFranchi SH: Hypothyroidism. Pediatr Clin North Am 26:33–51, 1979

Frasier SD: Growth disorders in children. Pediatr Clin North Am 26:1–14, 1979

* See Glossary

Gardner LI: Endocrine and Genetic Diseases of Childhood and Adolescence. Philadelphia, W. B. Saunders, 1975

Golden MP: An approach to the management of obesity in childhood. Pediatr Clin North Am 26:187–189, 1979

Kaplan SA: Diseases of the adrenal cortex II. Congenital adrenal hyperplasia. Pediatr Clin North Am 26:77–89, 1979

Lee WNP: Thyroiditis, hyperthyroidism, and tumors. Pediatr Clin North Am 26:53–64, 1979

Merrin C: Seminoma. Urol Clin North Am 4:379–3921, 1977

Munro DS et al: Thyroid-stimulating immunoglobulins and neonatal thyrotoxicosis. Br J Obstet Gynaecol 83:837–843, 1978

Sperling MA: Diabetes mellitus. Pediatr Clin North Am 26:149–169, 1979

Tsang RC, Noguchi A, Steichen JJ: Pediatric parathyroid disorders. Pediatr Clin North Am 26:223–249, 1979

Williams RH: Textbook of Endocrinology. Philadelphia, W. B. Saunders, 1974

12

Fluid and Electrolyte Therapy

GENERAL CONSIDERATIONS

A. Expenditure of water and electrolytes much greater per unit of body weight in children than in adults
B. Infants require 150–200 cc water/kg/day whereas adults require only 30–40 cc water/kg/day
C. Larger turnover of water in infants makes them particularly susceptible to development of dehydration and electrolyte imbalance. Because of this, conditions that cause excessive loss (*i.e.*, vomiting, diarrhea) or reduced intake require prompt treatment
D. Fluid therapy for treatment of dehydration and loss of electrolytes consists of *maintenance* (that required normally) plus *replacement* (that required to replace the losses that have occurred)

MAINTENANCE THERAPY

A. Calculated on basis of surface area, which may be obtained from standard nomograms. In general, the following surface areas relate to the following specific weights:
1. 10-kg infant–0.5m²
2. 30-kg child–1.0 m²
3. 60-kg person–1.5 m²
4. Average adult–1.7 m²

B. Normal requirements per square meter are as follows:
1. Water: 1500–2000 ml (750 ml during 1st week)
2. Sodium: 35–50 mEq (120 mEq during 1st week)
3. Potassium: 30–40 mEq (15 mEq during 1st week)

C. Normal saline contains about 150 mEq sodium per liter

REPLACEMENT THERAPY

A. Amount of Fluid
   Estimation of fluid loss
   a. Loss of fluid in dehydration ranges from 5% to 20%
   b. Mild dehydration = 5% loss
   c. Moderate dehydration = 10% loss
   d. Severe dehydration = 15–20% loss
      1. Children moribund from dehydration estimated to have 20% loss
      2. Only half of estimated fluid loss should be replaced during first 24 hours (attempts to replace *all* fluid loss can lead to water intoxication). Thus, replacement in *severe* dehydration is about 10% of body weight; in *moderate* dehydration, about 5%; and in *mild* dehydration, about 2.5%. Thus, a 10-kg, severely dehydrated child would receive 1000 ml of replacement fluid in first 24 hours

B. Type of Fluid
   In most cases, normal saline solution with added potassium if potassium deficiency exists. If acidosis is present, bicarbonate should be added (dose of bicarbonate is about 3 mEq/kg/12 hr)

C. Specific Deficiencies
   1. *Potassium* deficiency should not be corrected until urine flow is adequate
   2. *Calcium* deficiency should be suspected when increased irritability or seizures are present
   3. *Phosphorous* deficiency may exist in diabetic ketoacidosis

RATE OF ADMINISTRATION

A. If moribund or in state of collapse, isotonic saline, plasma, albumin solution, or blood used initially (20–30 ml/kg saline or plasma during first hour; 10–20 ml/kg blood during first hour)
B. One-fourth of total daily dose is given over each 6-hour period

DIAGNOSIS OF DEHYDRATION

A. Clinical Manifestations
   1. Loss of skin turgor
   2. Sunken eyes
   3. Depressed fontanelle
   4. Doughy skin, hyperirritability in hypernatremic dehydration
B. Laboratory Findings
   1. Plasma sodium normal (isonatremic dehydration), decreased (hyponatremic dehydration), or increased (hypernatremic dehydration). Isonatremic dehydration is most common
   2. Elevated BUN and serum creatinine

HYPERNATREMIC DEHYDRATION

General Considerations
1. Occurs particularly with acute diarrhea in infancy
2. Should be suspected if skin is doughy, warm, and dry
3. Nuchal rigidity and positive Kernig sign often present
4. Extreme irritability, restlessness, convulsions may be present
5. Amount of saline solution in these cases should *never* exceed 5% of body weight and should be given as 0.2% saline (30 mEq Na/liter) for mild dehydration and ⅓ N saline (50 mEq Na/liter) for moderate dehydration. If amount of dehydration exceeds 10%, remainder of fluid requirement should be made up with 5% dextrose in distilled water

BIBLIOGRAPHY

Kaplan SA: Fluid and electrolyte therapy: Maintenance, abnormal states, methods of administration. Pediatr Clin North Am 16:581–591, 1969

Rudolph AM, Barnett HL, Einhorn AH: Pediatrics. New York, Appleton-Century-Crofts, 1977

13

Pediatric Gynecology

MENSTRUAL DISORDERS

A. Normal Puberty
   1. Breast hypertrophy usually first sign (about 8–13 years)
   2. Pubic hair commonly comes next
   3. Axillary hair follows
   4. Menstruation last sign
   5. Breast development precedes menstruation by about 2 years
B. Amenorrhea
   1. Definition
      a. Absence or abnormal cessation of menses
      b. May be primary (onset of menses never occurred) or secondary (cessation of menses after normal onset)
   2. Etiology
      a. Defect in hormonal control or anatomic deficiency of genital organs
      b. Tumors of hypothalamus
         Rare
      c. Testicular feminization syndrome, vaginal atresia, imperforate hymen

      d. Congenital adrenal hyperplasia if untreated

      e. Hypothyroidism

3. Primary amenorrhea

    a. Normal secondary sexual development

        Generally due to anatomic defect

         a. Imperforate hymen: Usually presents with low abdominal pain, urinary difficulty, distended vagina with bulging bluish membrane

         b. Atresia of vagina: Diagnosis by physical examination. Buccal smear excludes testicular feminization (androgen insensitivity). Intravenous pyelogram indicated for detection of urinary tract anomalies (frequently present). Laparoscopy or ultrasound necessary to confirm absence of uterus

         c. Blind vagina: Confirmed by physical examination. Absence of uterus and cervix suggests testicular feminization syndrome.* Patient with buccal smear negative for nuclear chromatin should have chromosome analysis on peripheral blood to confirm XY karyotype

    b. Poor secondary sexual development

       1. Generally due to poor or absent gonadotropin production or failure of ovary to respond to gonadotropin

       2. Most prominent ovarian cause is gonadal dysgenesis (Turner's syndrome)

       3. Differentiation of pituitary versus ovarian defect by urine assay of gonadotropin (decreased in pituitary defect, increased in ovarian defect)

       4. Karyotype should be performed

    c. Bisexual development

       1. Masculinization with retarded female secondary sexual development

       2. May be variant of gonadal dysgenesis, congenital adrenal hyperplasia, androgen-producing tumor of adrenal gland or ovary

       3. Buccal smear and chromosomal analysis indicated (normal female karyotype consistent with congenital adrenal hyperplasia)

       4. Urinalysis for 17-oxysteroids

    d. Treatment

       1. Imperforate hymen requires surgical incision

       2. Absence of vagina requires surgical reconstruction

       3. Tumors require surgery and possibly chemotherapy

4. Secondary amenorrhea

    a. Gaps of about 3–6 months during first 10 menstrual cycles are normal

    b. Disturbances of hypothalamus and pituitary are frequently to blame

    c. Crash diet, emotional disturbances, anorexia nervosa, discontinuance of birth control pill, premature ovarian failure, chronic active hepatitis can also be causes

    d. Patient with brief duration of amenorrhea who is in good health may require psychosocial evaluation

---

* See Glossary

é. If prolonged, peripheral blood hemogram, urinary gonadotropins and adrenal steroids, skull roentgenogram of pituitary fossa, serum thyroid hormones, and visual field test are indicated

f. Spontaneous recovery occurs in the majority

g. Treatment directed at underlying problem

5. Oligomenorrhea
   a. Generally normal
   b. Can be reflection of anorexia, anemia, hypothalamic disorder, Stein-Leventhal syndrome (see hirsutism)
   c. Presence of hirsution or androgen excess indicates endocrine dysfunction
   d. Usually no treatment required
   e. Can give oral contraceptive to regularize menstrual cycle
   f. Treat underlying condition

6. Dysfunctional uterine bleeding (polymenorrhea, dysmenorrhea)
   a. Polymenorrhea
      1. Irregular profuse bleeding
      2. May be prolonged bleeding or shortened cycle
      3. Important causes are missed abortion, tubal pregnancy, endocrine disorders, uterine and vaginal conditions
      4. Treat with oral contraceptives
   b. Dysmenorrhea (painful period)
      1. Most frequent cause of pelvic pain in adolescent female
      2. Rarely caused by organic disease
      3. Pain may start before, at onset, or during menstruation
      4. May be associated with nausea, vomiting, diarrhea, headache, breast tenderness, fatigue, irritability
      5. Cause unknown
      6. Treatment
         a. Analgesics (narcotics to be avoided), prostaglandin inhibitors
         b. Oral contraceptives
         c. Surgical dilation of cervical os (for severe cases)

VENEREAL DISEASES

A. Gonococcal Infections
   1. Caused by Neisseria gonorrhoeae
   2. About 80–90% are asymptomatic
   3. Cervicitis
      Presenting complaints are discharge, dysuria, urinary frequency, painful intercourse
   4. Proctitis
      Occasionally seen
   5. Pharyngitis
      Sore throat, inflamed soft palate and tonsilar pillars

6. Vulvovaginitis
   a. Usually purulent discharge
   b. Child abuse must be considered in young patient
7. Pelvic inflammatory disease
   a. Primarily caused by gonococcus
   b. May be caused by Chlamydia trachomatis, staphylococci, anaerobic bacteria
   c. Infection results from spread of cervicitis to uterus and fallopian tubes during menses
   d. Usually presents with acute lower abdominal pain, fever, chills, vaginal discharge
   e. May be associated with menstrual irregularities, vomiting, diarrhea, or constipation, dysuria
   f. Can cause scarring of tubes with infertility, pelvic abscess
8. Arthritis
   Two forms
   1. *Early onset:* Just at or after menses. Presents with migratory polyarthralgias, tenosynovitis, fever, chills, skin lesions
   2. *Late onset:* Monoarticular swelling, pain, and tenderness
9. Endocarditis and meningitis are rare
10. Diagnosis
    a. Blood, joint fluid, vaginal, pharyngeal, rectal cultures and Gram stains
    b. Clinical signs and symptoms
11. Treatment
    a. Outpatient penicillin for localized disease
    b. Hospitalization with penicillin therapy for systemic infection

B. Syphilis
   1. Incidence increasing
   2. Stages of syphilis
      a. *Primary:* Presents about 10–90 days after sexual contact with painless chancre of vulva, vagina, cervix, or mouth. Inguinal adenopathy may be present. Serologic test may take 5–6 weeks to become positive
      b. *Secondary:* If chancre untreated, patient may get maculopapular rash (usually palms and soles), fever, malaise, hair loss, lymphadenopathy, venereal warts (condylomata lata) 6 weeks to several months later. Serum VDRL always positive
      c. *Latent:* Asymptomatic. May be infectious and may develop symptoms of tertiary syphilis
      d. *Tertiary:* Presence of gummas,* neurologic and cardiovascular disorders
   3. Treatment
      Varying amounts of penicillin depending on stage of disease

C. Trichomonas Vaginalis
   1. Presents as acute yellow discharge and red vaginal epithelium. Can be mistaken for cystitis

* Glossary

    2. Many infections result in asymptomatic carriers

    3. Diagnosis by microscopic examination of discharge

D. Chlamydia Trachomatis

    1. Cause of significant number of nonspecific infections and pelvic inflammatory disease (salpingitis)

    2. Nonspecific infection can present with sterile discharge without accompanying symptoms

    3. Salpingitis presents with chills, fever, myalgia, anorexia, nausea, vomiting, lower abdominal pain

       Tubular obstruction with resulting infertility complicates disease

    4. Tetracycline for nonspecific infection

    5. No treatment for salpingitis

E. Herpes Simplex Type II

    1. Initial symptoms are pruritis, irritation

    2. Later developments include vesicles and ulceration of vulva, vaginal wall, cervix

    3. Primary infection produces severe pain in genital area, fever

    4. Associated with cervical cancer

    5. Effective treatment not available

CONTRACEPTIVES

A. Condoms

    1. For teenager most easily available and cheap

    2. Protects against venereal disease

B. Spermicidal Creams, Jellies, Foams

    1. Produce spermicidal environment in vagina

    2. Must be inserted no more than 60 minutes before intercourse

    3. Foam most effective

    4. Pregnancy rate about 6%

    5. Combination of condom and foam more effective

C. Diaphragm

    1. Very effective

    2. Rare side effects

    3. Used with spermicidal jelly or cream

    4. Must be fitted by physician

D. Rhythm Method

    1. To be most effective, cycle should be charted for 1 year

    2. Irregularity of adolescent and ignorance make this method ineffective in this age group

E. Douching

    No value

F. Intrauterine Device (IUD)

    1. Highly effective method of contraception

2. Must be inserted by physician
3. Regular physical examination by physician advised
4. Complications include excessive bleeding, pain, pregnancy with IUD still in cervix, expulsion of IUD, pelvic inflammatory disease, perforation of uterus

G. Oral Contraceptives
1. Preferred by many adolescents because of low failure rate and marked lessening of dysmenorrhea
2. Combination pills frequently prescribed
    Suppress ovulation and implantation
3. Complications
    a. Nausea, bloating, weight gain, headaches
    b. Hypertension (in about 5%)
        Contraindicated in hypertensive individuals
    c. Thrombophlebitis
    d. Abnormal glucose tolerance test
    e. Abnormal liver function tests occasionally with jaundice
4. Contraindications
    a. Collagen vascular disease (lupus erythematosis, rheumatoid arthritis)
    b. Recent hepatitis or cholestatic jaundice

HIRSUTISM

A. Definition
1. Excessive growth of sexual hair (pubic, axillary, abdominal, chest, facial areas) in female with or without signs of virilization
2. Excessive hair growth manifested by coarseness, longer length than is normal for age, sex, race

B. Incidence
1. Common in adolescent female
2. About half of women with hirsutism present under 20 years of age

C. History and Physical Examination
1. Date of onset, progression and duration of disorder, presence and duration of associated symptoms
2. Past childhood diseases and menstrual history plus current medication record
3. Degree and distribution of hirsutism should be noted
4. Presence of defeminization (regression of breast size) and virilization (male muscular pattern, enlargement of clitoris, acne, voice change) should be noted

D. Etiology
1. May be related to race, family tendency
2. Iatrogenic hirsutism
    a. *Trauma:* Hirsutism may occur transiently after skin trauma inflicted by friction or intermittent pressure (casts)
    b. *Drugs:* Phenytoin (Dilantin), steroids, hexachlorobenzene, diazoxide, cobalt can cause hirsutism with or without virilization. Hair growth typi-

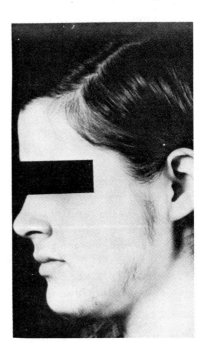

Fig. 82. Hirsutism in an adolescent with Stein-Levanthal syndrome. (*Leng JJ, Greenblatt RB: Hirsutism in adolescent girls. Pediatr Clin North Am 19:681, 1972*)

cally occurs 2–3 months after initial therapy. Hair on extensor surface of extremities or trunk and face commonly affected

3. Central nervous system
   a. Can occur secondary to cerebral trauma or infection
   b. Chronic disease, starvation
4. Endocrinopathies
   a. Adrenals
      1. Congenital adrenal hyperplasia (if untreated)
      2. Adrenocortical tumors (virilizing type). Removal causes return to normal if no metastases present
      3. Cushing's syndrome (rare in adolescents)
   b. Ovary
      1. *Stein-Leventhal syndrome:* Hirsutism, normal breast development, obesity, menstrual dysfunction (oligomenorrhea or amenorrhea), multicystic ovaries (Fig. 82). Ovary thought to be source of androgens. Treat with combination oral contraceptives to restore regular menses and suppress ovary. Bilateral wedge resections to restore normal ovulatory cycle usually not done in adolescent
      2. *Tumors of ovary (virilizing):* Infrequently seen in adolescent. Presents with regression of female secondary sexual development and virilization
   c. Thyroid
      Hypothyroidism

      d. Pituitary

          Hyperplasia of anterior pituitary

   5. Associated with abnormal sexual development

      a. Male pseudohermaphroditism

      b. Gonadal dysgenesis with abdominal testes

   6. Congenital anomalies

      a. Trisomy 18 (see Chap. XXI)

      b. Hurler's syndrome (see Chap. XXIII)

   7. Idiopathic

E. Diagnosis

   1. Clinical signs and symptoms

   2. Urine assay for 17-ketosteroids

   3. Dexamethasone test (should be done if urinary 17-ketosteroids are elevated)

      a. Elevation of urine 17-ketosteroids despite suppression of cortisol by dexamethasone is suspicious of adrenal or ovarian tumor

      b. Lowering of urine 17-ketosteroids suggests congenital adrenal hyperplasia

F. Treatment

      Treat underlying condition

AMBIGUOUS GENITALIA (see Fig. 78)

A. Embryology

   1. Development of gonad into testicle dependent on presence of Y chromosome

   2. Need at least two X chromosomes for normal ovary

   3. At eighth fetal week, both müllerian and wolffian gonaducts are present

   4. Absence of testes with their inducer substances causes regression of wolffian structures

   5. External genitalia masculinize due to androgen secreted by fetal Leydig cells

B. Studies

   1. *Buccal smear:* Positive if two X chromosomes present

   2. Karyotyping of peripheral smear

C. Pseudohermaphrodite

   1. Female

      a. Presence of ovaries with ambiguous external genitalia

      b. Caused by excess fetal or maternal androgen (*i.e.,* virilizing ovarian tumor, ingestion of androgen, congenital adrenal hyperplasia)

      c. Congenital virilizing adrenal hyperplasia most common cause

      d. Physical examination reveals labioscrotal fusion, clitoral enlargement

      e. Most often labia majora appear as bifid scrotum with urogenital sinus evident at base of phallus

   2. Male

      a. Presence of testes with ambiguous external genitalia

      b. Can present as near normal male (perineal hypospadius) to normal appearing female (testicular feminization)

c. Testes can be present in abdomen, inguinal canal, or labioscrotal folds

d. Buccal smears are indicated when gonads can be palpated in inguinal canal in presence of external female genitalia

D. True Hermaphrodite

1. Presence of testis and ovary
2. True pathogenesis not understood
3. Karyotypes reveal mosaics and varying abnormal numbers of sex chromosomes
4. Treatment directed at surgical construction most consistent with external appearance

BIBLIOGRAPHY

Colodny AH, Hopkins TB: Testicular tumors in infants and children. Urol Clin North Am 4:347–358, 1977

Dewhurst CJ: Amenorrhea and the paediatrician. Pediatr Clin North Am 19:605–618, 1972

Emans SJH, Goldstein DP: Pediatric and Adolescent Gynecology. Boston, Little, Brown, 1977

Grodin JM: Secondary amenorrhea in the adolescent. Pediatr Clin North Am 19:619–630, 1972

Leng JJ, Greenblatt, RB: Hirsutism in adolescent girls. Pediatr Clin North Am 19:681–703, 1972

Lippe BM: Ambiguous genitalia and pseudohermaphroditism. Pediatr Clin North Am 26:77–89, 1979

Marinoff SC: Contraception in adolescents. Pediatr Clin North Am 19:811–819, 1972

Nochomovitz LE, DeLaTorre FE, Rosai J: Pathology of germ cell tumors of the testis. Urol Clin North Am 4:359–378, 1977

14

Common Pediatric Skin Disorders

MILIARIA CRYSTALLINA (Fig. 83)

General Considerations
1. Common lesions in immediate newborn period resulting from sweat retention
2. 1–2 mm in diameter, usually on forehead, upper trunk, arms
3. Disappear spontaneously

ERYTHEMA TOXICUM (see Fig. 6)

General Considerations
1. Occurs during first week of life
2. Blotchy maculopapular erythema
3. May be limited or widespread
4. Benign and self-limited

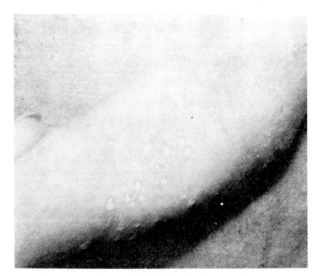

Fig. 83. Discrete lesions of miliaria crystallina on the arm in a term infant at 48 hours. Note the clear fluid content and absence of inflammation. (*Hodgman JE et al: Neonatal dermatology. Pediatr Clin North Am 18:713, 1971*)

VASCULAR NEVI

A. Nevus Simplex (salmon patch, Fig. 84)
    1. Very common in newborn
    2. Red macular lesion on nape of neck ("stork bite"), upper eyelids, nasolabial area
    3. Majority fade during first year of life
B. Nevus Flammeus (port-wine stain, Fig. 85)
    1. Red to purple in color, not elevated
    2. Present from birth on
    3. Variable in size, shape, location
    4. May be component of Sturge-Weber syndrome
    5. Is a capillary hemangioma

NEVUS VASCULOSIS
(STRAWBERRY HEMANGIOMA) (Fig. 86)

General Considerations
1. May appear as early as 2–3 days of life but not at birth
2. A capillary hemangioma
3. Resembles strawberry in appearance (raised, red, rough, sharply demarcated
4. Occurs anywhere but usually on head and neck
5. Majority undergo gradual regression and disappear by 5–10 years of age

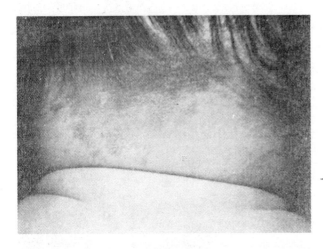

Fig. 84. Nevus simplex of the neck. In this location, the lesion is commonly called a "stork bite." One that persists is known as Unna's nevus. (*Hodgman JE et al: Neonatal dermatology. Pediatr Clin North Am 18:713, 1971*)

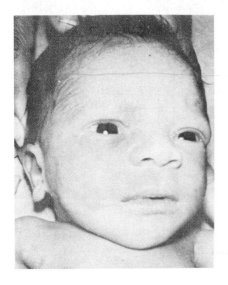

Fig. 85. Port-wine stain in the distribution of the trigeminal nerve. Infants with nevus flammeus in this distrubition must have additional studies to rule out Sturge-Weber syndrome. (*Hodgman JE et al: Neonatal dermatology. Pediatr Clin North Am 18:713, 1971*)

CAVERNOUS HEMANGIOMAS

General Considerations
1. Collection of vessels with bluish but normal overlying skin
2. Present at birth
3. Affected area is large and distorted
4. Vary in size and location
5. If large, arteriovenous shunts may cause heart failure
6. Coagulopathy with thrombocytopenia may result from sequestration of platelets
7. Some may regress spontaneously

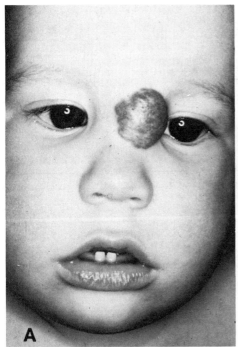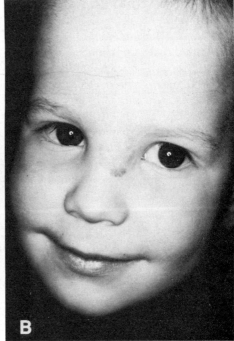

Fig. 86. Strawberry hemangioma. **(A)** Lesion at its greatest size. **(B)** Same lesion 26 months later, without treatment. (*McGuire J: In Rudolph AM, Barnett HL, Einhorn AH (eds): Pediatrics, p 901. New York, Appleton-Century-and Crofts, 1977*)

8. Some require systemic corticosteroid therapy
9. Extensive involvement not responding to steroids may require surgical excision

UMBILICAL GRANULOMA

General Considerations
1. Umbilical cord dries and usually separates about a week after birth
2. Occasionally, mild infection results in moist granulating area at base of cord after separation
3. Mucoid or mucopurulent discharge present
4. Red granulation tissue persists
5. Responds readily to daily alcohol cleansing and cauterization with silver nitrate

MONGOLIAN SPOTS

See Chapter 2, page 9.

DIAPER RASH (AMMONIACAL DERMATITIS)

General Considerations
1. Is a contact or chemical dermatitis due to ammonia in urine
2. Eruption is parchmentlike erythema in diaper area with creases spared
3. In males, meatal ulcer may be associated
4. Responds promptly to treatment
    a. Expose area to air as much as possible
    b. Change diapers frequently
    c. Eliminate impervious diaper covers
    d. Instruct mother *not* to double diaper
    e. Topical glucocorticoid cream (*avoid oily* or *greasy* preparations)

CANDIDIASIS IN DIAPER AREA (MONILIA)
(FIG. 87)

General Considerations
1. Often follows oral thrush
2. Moist intertrigo (inflammatory process in folds) with satellite lesions
3. May be primary in perianal region
4. Responds to nystatin dusting powder

SEBORRHEIC DERMATITIS (FIG. 88)

General Considerations
1. Common in infants particularly on scalp ("cradle cap") or in diaper area complicating ammoniacal dermatitis
2. Yellowish crusts on scalp
3. Sharply demarcated eczematous rash in diaper area
4. Self-limited but responds readily to topical glucocorticoid cream

INSECT BITES

General Considerations
1. Local reactions resulting from bites of many kinds of insects (mosquitoes and fleas most common)
2. Characteristic response is evanescent, urticarial papule with marked pruritis
3. Response may be chronic, recurrent, and papulovesicular in appearance (papular urticaria, Fig. 89)
4. Treatment consists of protection from or elimination of source

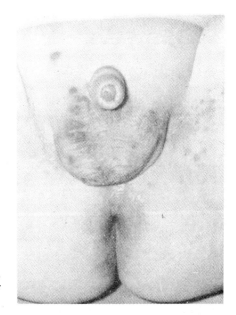

Fig. 87. Perianal candidiasis with satellite lesions. (*Jacobs AH: Eruptions in the diaper area. Pediatr Clin North Am 25:209, 1978*)

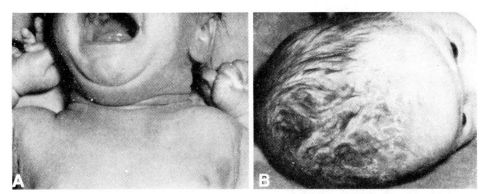

Fig. 88. (A) Seborrheic dermatitis involving the axillae and neck folds. **(B)** Cradle cap due to seborrheic dermatitis. (*Jacobs AH: Eruptions in the diaper area. Pediatr Clin North Am 25:209, 1978*)

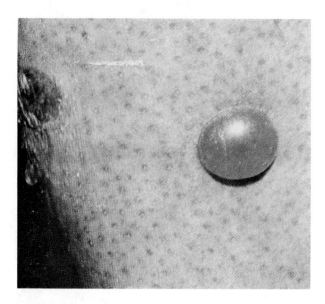

Fig. 89. Bullous reaction to mosquito bite. (*Korting GW, Curth W, Curth HO: Diseases of the Skin in Children and Adolescents. A Color Atlas, p 89. Philadelphia, W. B. Saunders, 1970*)

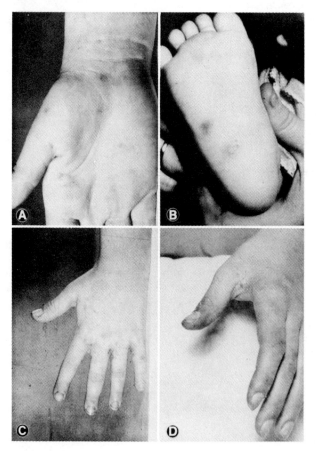

Fig. 90. Scabies in children. Note the palmar **(A)**, plantar **(B)**, and web locations **(C,D)** of the burrows. (*From the collection of the Skin and Cancer Unit of the New York University Hospital.*) (*From Leider M: Practical Pediatric Dermatology, p 192. Saint Louis, C. V. Mosby, 1961*)

SCABIES (FIG. 90)

General Considerations
1. Caused by *Sarcoptes scabiei* mite
2. Characterized by pruritic papulovesicular eruption particularly in interdigital areas, palms, body folds, genital area
3. Pruritis more marked at night
4. Diagnosis confirmed by demonstration of mite in a skin burrow (tiny straight or tortuous linear elevation)
5. May be complicated by secondary infection
6. Treatment consists of application of local scabicides (*lindane,* not to be used in infants and young children because of possible absorption with central nervous system toxicity; crotamiton; sulfur preparations; gamma benzene hexachloride (*Kwell*), not to be used in infants and young children because of possible absorption and toxicity)

WARTS

General Considerations
1. Small benign tumors of skin occurring in preschool, school-age children, adolescents
2. Due to a specific viral agent (papovavirus)
3. Occur most commonly on hands, forearms, soles of feet (plantar warts)
4. Usually resolve spontaneously within 2 years but plantar warts can be painful and may require treatment

IMPETIGO CONTAGIOSUM (FIG. 91)

General Considerations
1. Superficial skin infection caused by beta-hemolytic streptococcus or Staphylococcus aureus
2. Vesicles or pustules that become exudative and crusted
3. Face is most common location
4. Bullous impetigo common in first few weeks of life
   a. Usually occurs in diaper area
   b. Due to Staphylococcus aureus
   c. Treatment consists of carefully debriding bullae and application of bacitracin ointment. Antistaphylococcal antibiotics may be indicated
5. May be complicated by glomerulonephritis (due to nephritogenic strains of streptococci)
6. Treatment
   a. Gentle removal of crusts using water and hexachlorophene
   b. Cleansing with hexachlorophene
   c. Penicillin therapy with extensive involvement

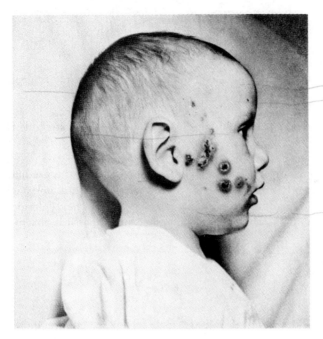

Fig. 91. Impetigo. (*Radcliffe CE: In Top FH (ed): Communicable and Infectious Diseases. Diagnosis, Prevention, Treatment. Saint Louis, C. V. Mosby, 1964*)

ACNE VULGARIS

A. General Considerations
   1. Most common skin disorder in adolescents
   2. Characterized by follicular obstruction with secondary infection
   3. Related to many factors including androgen excess, increased sebum excretion rate, heredity
   4. Type of diet probably not a factor
B. Manifestations
   1. Lesions include comedones ("blackheads"), inflammatory papules, pustules, nodules, cysts, scars
   2. Most prominent on face but may occur on back, chest, upper arms, thighs, buttocks
C. Treatment
   1. Local application of retinoic acid, benzoyl peroxide, sulfur preparations
   2. Ultraviolet light
   3. Mechanical drainage of comedones and superficial pustules
   4. Nodules not to be incised and drained since this may result in permanent scarring
   5. Systemic antibacterials with tetracycline as first choice
D. Course
   A chronic lingering disease but therapy may result in slow (but steady) improvement

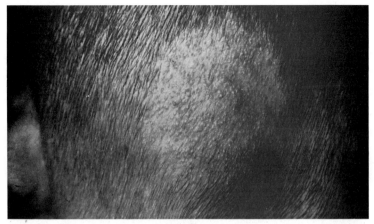

Fig. 92. Tinea capitis. Etiologic agent was *Microsporum audouini.* (*Sauer GC: Manual of Skin Diseases, 3rd ed. Philadelphia, J. B. Lippincott, 1973*)

FUNGAL INFECTIONS

A. Timea Capitis (scalp ringworm, Fig. 92)
  1. May have crusts, silvery scales, edematous inflammation of scalp (kerion), alopecia
  2. Treatment consists of daily shampoo, oral griseofulvin, oral prednisone, broad-spectrum antibiotic if secondarily infected

B. Tinea Corporis (Fig. 93)
  1. Lesions vary from dry scaling to weeping vesicular dermatitis
  2. Lesions usually annular
  3. Diagnosis confirmed by microscopic demonstration of mycelia in KOH preparation of scales. Also by culture
  4. Treatment consists of local application of fungicides such as tolnaftate (Tinactin), clotrimazole (Lotrimin), haloprogin (Halotex)

C. Tinea Cruris ("jock-strap itch")
  1. Erythematous lesions with serpiginous border in upper thigh area
  2. Diagnosis by KOH preparation and culture
  3. Treatment as for *Tinea corporis*

D. Tinea Pedis (athlete's foot)
  1. Most commonly in intertriginous area between fourth and fifth toes. Often extends to adjacent toes and arch of foot
  2. Characterized by skin desquamation, pruritis. In severe cases may get vesicles, pustules, weeping crusts
  3. Treatment
    a. Local debridement
    b. Exposure to air and sunlight
    c. Local application of fungicides

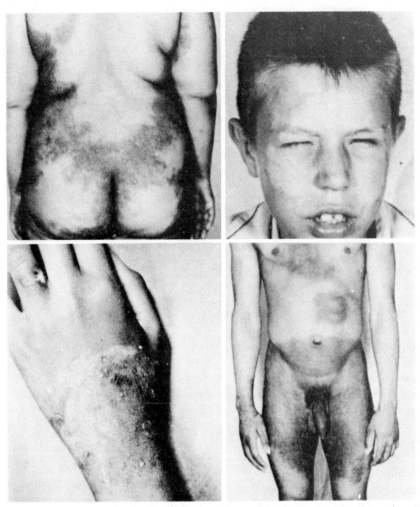

Fig. 93. Tinea corporis showing varied portions of body involved by these der-
matophytes. The etiologic agent isolated in the boy **(upper right)** was *Trichophyton
tonsurans*. (*Moss ES, McQuown AL: Atlas of Medical Mycology, p 207. Baltimore,
Williams & Wilkins, 1960*)

E. Tinea Versicolor
1. Circumscribed scaly lesions (darker or lighter than surrounding normal skin)
2. Commonly occur on upper trunk
3. Treatment by local application of haloprogin (Halotex), tolnaftate (Tinactin),
   selenium sulfide (Selsun), Tinver Lotion (sodium thiosulfate, salicylic acid,
   isopropyl alcohol)

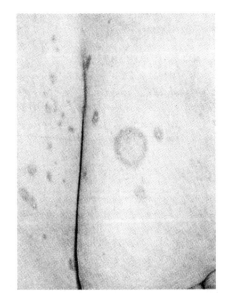

Fig. 94. Pityriasis rosea with typical herald patch (primary plaque). (*Korting GW, Curth W, Curth HO: Diseases of the Skin in Children and Adolescents. A Color Atlas, p 23. Philadelphia, W. B. Saunders, 1970*)

PITYRIASIS ALBA

General Considerations
1. Probably an early variant of atopic dermatitis
2. Lesions are dry, scaly, hypopigmented
3. Commonly involves cheeks, upper back, upper arms
4. Does not respond to treatment
5. Self-limited disease with disappearance usually in 2–3 years

PITYRIASIS ROSEA

General Considerations
1. Characterized by pinkish, oval scaling lesions
2. Mostly on trunk
3. Probably infectious in origin
4. First sign is solitary lesion that enlarges and clears centrally ("herald lesion," Fig. 94)
5. Multiple similar but smaller lesions occur within 1–2 weeks
6. May be pruritic
7. Disease is self-limited with spontaneous disappearance of lesions in 4–6 weeks

HERPES LABIALIS ("COLD SORE," "FEVER BLISTER")

General Considerations
1. Caused by herpes simplex
2. Painful vesicles with erosion and crusting on lips. Also involves tongue, palate, gingiva, buccal mucosa
3. May be associated with fever and toxicity
4. Periodic localized recurrences on vermilion border of lip common
5. Recurrent lesions heal spontaneously and are not associated with toxicity

BIBLIOGRAPHY

Arundell FD: Acne vulgaris. Pediatr Clin North Am 18:853–874, 1971

Goldberg MP: The oral mucosa in childhood. Pediatr Clin North Am 25:239–262, 1978

Hodgman JE, Freedman RI, Levan NE: Neonatal dermatology. Pediatr Clin North Am 18:713–756, 1971

Jacobs AH: Eruptions in the diaper area. Pediatr Clin North Am 25:209–224, 1978

Jacobs PH: Fungal infections in childhood. Pediatr Clin North Am 25:357–370, 1978

Koblenzer PJ: Common bacterial infections of the skin in children. Pediatr Clin North Am 25:321–338, 1978

Margileth AM: Developmental vascular abnormalities. Pediatr Clin North Am 18:773–779, 1971

Moss EM: Atopic dermatitis. Pediatr Clin North Am 25:225–238, 1978

Orkin M, Maibach HI: Scabies in children. Pediatr Clin North Am 25:371–386, 1978

15

Common Allergic Disorders

URTICARIA (HIVES)

A. Definition

Well-circumscribed wheals or welts of various sizes. May coalesce into large lesions (giant hives). An IgE-mediated allergy. Associated with intense pruritis.

B. Incidence

1. Common, as high as 20% of population at one time or another
2. More frequent in females

C. Etiology

1. *Ingestants* (particularly shellfish, nuts, chocolate, eggs, drugs)
2. *Contactants* (drugs, animal saliva, plants)
3. *Injectants* (drugs, insect bites and stings, blood transfusions)
4. *Inhalants* (pollens, molds, danders)
5. *Infection* (parasitic infestations)

D. Treatment

a. Usually self-limited
b. Sometimes recurrent and chronic

    c. Epinephrine gives rapid relief

    d. Antihistamines

ATOPIC ECZEMA

A. Manifestations
1. In infants, erythematous, weeping, crusty patches on face (*infantile eczema*)
2. Flexural areas (popliteal and antecubital) may become involved but usually at later age (neurodermatitis)
3. Onset often coincides with introduction of certain foods (*i.e.*, cow's milk, wheat, eggs)
4. Generally runs course in 1–5 years

B. Diagnosis
1. Family history of allergic disease
2. Clinical manifestations

C. Treatment
1. Avoidance of suspected cause
2. Avoidance of temperature extremes
3. Avoidance of wool or abrasive clothing
4. Infrequent bathing with avoidance of soaps and detergents
5. Local therapy (wet dressings, corticosteroid creams)
6. Systemic antibiotics for infection
7. Antihistamines, particularly diphenhydramine hydrochloride (Benadryl) (because of its sedative effect)
8. Elbow restraints, short finger nails (to prevent trauma from scratching)
9. With severe involvement resistant to treatment, systematic corticosteroids may be indicated

BRONCHIAL ASTHMA

A. General Considerations
1. A leading cause of chronic disease in childhood
2. A diffuse obstructive disease of small and large airways that can usually be reversed with appropriate treatment
3. Prolonged symptoms not responding to epinephrine termed "status asthmaticus"
4. Is a complex disorder involving infection, psychologic and endocrine as well as immunologic factors
5. Attacks may follow exposure to dust, pollens, and danders and be precipitated by respiratory infections

B. Manifestations
1. Insidious or abrupt onset
2. Wheezing, cough, prolonged expiration, dyspnea, apprehension, sweating, fatigue

    3. May be complicated by atelectasis, pneumothorax, pneumomediastinum

    4. Severe chronic cases may be complicated by emphysema

    5. Episodes tend to be recurrent

C. Diagnosis

    1. Characteristic clinical manifestations

    2. Relief with epinephrine therapy

D. Treatment

    1. Avoidance of allergens

    2. Hyposensitization

    3. For acute attacks, epinephrine, epinephrine hydrochloride (Sus-Phrine), theophylline. In status asthmaticus, add isoproterenol, corticosteroids, oxygen

    4. Theophylline, ephedrine, aerosolized isoproterenol, and if necessary, corticosteroids as maintenance therapy for severe recurrent cases

    5. Status asthmaticus requires hospitalization

ALLERGIC RHINITIS

A. General Considerations

    1. May be seasonal or perennial

    2. House dust, pollens, molds, danders often implicated

B. Manifestations

    1. Sneezing (often paroxysmal)

    2. *Watery,* profuse rhinorrhea

    3. Nasal obstruction

    4. Itching of nose, palate

    5. Itching, redness, tearing of eyes

    6. Cough

    7. Bluish boggy nasal mucosa

    8. Rubbing nose in upward direction ("allergic salute," Fig. 95)

    9. Wrinkling movements of nose ("rabbit nose")

   10. Horizontal crease on distal portion of nose ("allergic crease") as a consequence of upward rubbing (Fig. 96)

C. Diagnosis

    1. Family history

    2. History of allergic diathesis

    3. Manifestations

    4. Predominance of eosinophilia on nasal smear

D. Treatment

    1. Avoidance of offending agents

    2. Hyposensitization

    3. Antihistamines

E. Complications

    1. Increased susceptibility to upper respiratory infections and otitis media

    2. Nasal polyps

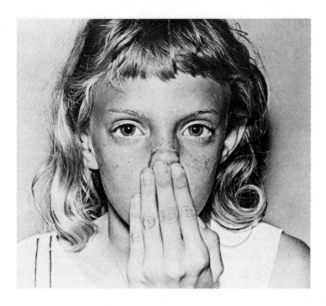

Fig. 95. The allergic salute induces transverse nasal crease. (*Marks MB, Stigmata of Respiratory Tract Allergies, p 12. Kalamazoo, Upjohn, 1972*)

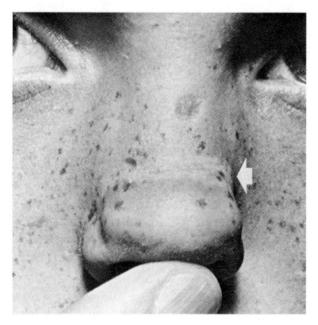

Fig. 96. Transverse nasal crease indicated by **arrow.** At least two years of pronounced "saluting" occurs before crease becomes ingrained. (*Marks MB: Stigmata of Respiratory Tract Allergies, p 13. Kalamazoo, Upjohn, 1972*)

F. Course
   1. Usually prolonged
   2. Not as likely as asthma to resolve spontaneously with age

ANGIONEUROTIC EDEMA

General Considerations
   1. Rare, recurrent disease characterized by recurrent swelling of face (particularly lips). Larynx may become edematous with resultant laryngeal obstruction and croup
   2. Usually allergic in nature
   3. May be associated with urticaria
   4. May respond to epinephrine, antihistamines
   5. Hereditary form due to deficiency of esterase inhibitor and is transmitted as an autosomal dominant
   6. Laryngeal involvement can be life-threatening

BIBLIOGRAPHY

Hoekelman RA et al: Principles of Pediatrics, Health Care of the Young. New York, McGraw-Hill, 1978

Rachelefsky GS: New drugs in the treatment of asthma. In Pediatrics Update. Reviews for Physicians, 1:304–326, 1979

Rudolph AM, Barnett HL, Einhorn AH: Pediatrics. New York, Appleton-Century-Crofts, 1977

Vaughan VC III, McKay RJ, Nelson WE: Nelson Textbook of Pediatrics. Philadelphia, W. B. Saunders, 1975

16

Immunologic Disorders

GENERAL CONSIDERATIONS

A. Development and Function of Immune System
1. Hematopoetic stem cells differentiate into thymus-dependent (T) and thymus-independent (B) lymphocytes
2. T lymphocytes are responsible for cell-mediated immunity (includes delayed hypersensitivity, graft rejection, graft-versus-host disease, immune protection against cancer, control of viral, fungal, and facultative intracellular infections)
3. Immune competence evidenced at 10–12 weeks of gestational age (cellular immunity)
4. Fetus can produce antibodies at 20th week of gestation (mainly IgM)
5. Infants begin forming IgG at end of second month. Adult levels achieved by end of first year

B. Classification
1. Antibody deficiency
   a. Most common primary immunodeficiency (50–75% of cases)
   b. Lack of IgA in serum and secretions is most common antibody deficiency

2. Cellular immunodeficiency
   a. Normal antibody production can be present (5–10% of cases)
   b. Combined cellular and antibody deficiency more common (10–25% of cases)
   c. Usually associated with thymic hypoplasia or dysplasia
3. Phagocytic immunodeficiencies
   a. Seen in about 17% of cases
   b. Anatomic anomalies (asplenia)
   c. Granulocytic disorders (chronic granulomatous disease)
4. Complement deficiency
   Occurs in less than 1% of cases
5. Immunodeficiency of immaturity
   a. Results in high rate of infection in early life
   b. Occurs particularly in premature infant
6. Secondary immunodeficiency
   Disease process that causes transitory or permanent immunoincompetence
C. Incidence
   1. Antibody deficiency occurs in about 1 per 100,000
   2. More common in males than females
D. Etiology
   1. Unknown
   2. Congenital rubella associated with IgG deficiency
   3. Several diseases have X-linked or autosomal recessive inheritance patterns
E. Manifestations
   1. Increased frequency of infection that is unusually severe and prolonged and is caused by organism of low pathogenicity
   2. Unexpected complications
   3. Past history of abnormal response to vaccinations, severe infections, no allergies
   4. Family history of relatives with similar problems
   5. Underdeveloped, pallor, distended abdomen, skin rashes, absence of tonsils and cervical lymph nodes, thrush, cheilosis often noted
   6. Respiratory infections
      a. Most common of all infections
      b. Streptococci, pneumococcus, Hemophilus influenzae most common bacteria
      c. Usually 6–8 infections per year (severe and sometimes complicated by pneumonia, bronchitis)
      d. Patient never completely recovers from previous illness
F. Evaluation of Immunocompetence
   1. *Antibody deficiency:* Hemogram, quantitative immunoglobulin levels, Schick test (evaluates IgG function), isoagglutinin titer (tests IgM function)
   2. *Cellular deficiency:* Chest film for thymic shadow, lymphocyte count on peripheral blood, skin tests (to determine presence of delayed hypersensitivity), in vitro studies of lymphocyte proliferation, transformation (lymphocyte activation by antigens)
   3. *Phagocytic defects:* Granulocyte count, nitroblue tetrazolium tests (tests phagocytizing ability of neutrophils)

G. Treatment
   1. Prevent congenital rubella, genetic counseling
   2. Remainder of treatment aimed at reducing infections
      a. Reduce exposure to pathogens
      b. No exercise restrictions
      c. Antibiotics for all infections
           Choice of drug same as for normal patient
      d. Human gamma globulin effective in cases of antibody deficiency; normal life span can be achieved
      e. Plasma (supplies IgG, IgM, IgA)
      f. Bone marrow transplantation
           May be effective in combined immunodeficiency

IMMUNODEFICIENCY OF IMMATURITY

Immunologic Responses of Fetus
1. Fetus can produce antibodies
2. Antibody production is absent or reduced due to acquired maternal antibodies that prevent antigenic stimulation
3. Antigenic stimulation *in utero* produces lymphoid hyperplasia and antibody production
4. Cellular immunity develops before birth
5. Homograft rejection occurs *in utero* in mammals
6. Fetal lymphocytes respond to phytohemagglutinin at end of first trimester
7. Factors suppressing neonatal antibody production
   a. Maternal antibodies
   b. Hyperbilirubinemia
8. Immunodeficiency in neonate
   a. All septic infants should be suspect
   b. Indications are maternal rubella infection, family history of infection with organisms of low virulence, unusual severity of disease
   c. Hemogram, quantitative immunoglobulins for IgM, phytohemagglutinin study of lymphocytes might help establish diagnosis
9. Transient hypogammaglobulinemia of infancy
   a. Self-limited
   b. Prolonged delay in gamma globulin production
   c. No recurrence after recovery
   d. Recover spontaneously by about 9–15 months
   e. Etiology unknown
   f. Especially prone to gram-positive bacterial infections of skin, lungs, meninges, respiratory tract
   g. Present with failure to thrive, continuous infections
   h. Diagnosis established by determination of quantitative immunoglobulins

i. Presence of plasma cells on rectal biopsy distinguishes this condition from X-linked agammaglobulinemia

j. Treatment consists of gamma globulin injections (if severe) and supportive care

ANTIBODY DEFICIENCY

A. General Considerations

May be associated with malabsorption, diarrhea, Giardia lamblia infections, autoimmune hemolytic anemia, neutropenia, thrombocytopenia, collagen vascular disease

B. Congenital Agammaglobulinemia (Bruton's agammaglobulinemia)

1. X-linked recessive
2. Well until about 6–12 months of age (probably because of maternal antibody protection)
3. Infections controlled by antibiotics
4. Absence of plasma cells in peripheral tissues

C. Selective Immunoglobulin Deficiency

1. IgA most common
   a. Usually asymptomatic
   b. Can be associated with steatorrhea, ulcerative colitis, Crohn's disease, atopy, collagen vascular disease
   c. May be familial
2. Selective deficiency of other globulins rare

CELLULAR IMMUNODEFICIENCY

A. General Considerations

1. Severe viral and fungal infections
2. Fatal BCG reaction and progressive illness following vaccination are important complications
3. Graft-versus-host disease after blood transfusion is important consideration

B. Thymic Hypoplasia (Di George Syndrome)

1. Failure of third and fourth pharyngeal pouches to develop
2. Aplasia of thymus and parathyroids
3. May be familial pattern
4. Presents as neonatal hypocalcemia
5. Associated defects are hypertelorism,* low-set ears, midline clefts, cardiac anomalies (right aortic arch, tetralogy of Fallot)
6. Cellular immunity impaired
7. Most often patient has incomplete form of disease that results in less severe course

Probably indicates hypoplasia and not aplasia

8. Thymic transplantation has resulted in cure

* See Glossary

COMBINED CELLULAR AND HUMORAL
IMMUNODEFICIENCY

A. Severe Combined Immunodeficiency Disease
   1. Most severe immune deficit
   2. Patient presents at about 3–9 months of age with recurrent disease, chronic diarrhea, candidiasis, failure to thrive
   3. Death usually before 2 years of age
   4. Autosomal recessive and X-linked pattern
B. Immunodeficiency with Eczema and Thrombocytopenia (Wiskott-Aldrich syndrome)
   1. X-linked recessive
   2. Initially, patient presents with bleeding
   3. Eczema, thrombocytopenia, recurrent infections seen later
   4. High association of lymphoreticular malignancy
   5. Disease characterized by progressive loss of cellular immunity and by low immunoglobulins (IgM)

BIBLIOGRAPHY

Hoekelman RA et al: Principles of Pediatrics, Health Care of the Young. New York, McGraw-Hill, 1978

Rudolph AM, Barnett HL, Einhorn AH: Pediatrics. New York, Appleton-Century-Crofts, 1977

Stiehm ER, Fulginiti VA: Immunologic Disorders in Infants and Children. Philadelphia, W. B. Saunders, 1973

Vaughan VC III, McKay RJ, Nelson WE: Nelson Textbook of Pediatrics. Philadelphia, W. B. Saunders, 1975

17 | Collagen–Vascular Diseases

MUCOCUTANEOUS LYMPH NODE SYNDROME (KAWASAKI DISEASE)

A. Etiology and Epidemiology
   1. Etiology unknown
   2. Mainly affects children under 5 years
B. Manifestations
   1. Erythema of conjunctivae, mucous membranes, and extremities. Edema, maculopopular rash, desquamation (especially of fingers), anterior cervical lymphadenopathy
   2. Thrombocytosis, elevated leukocyte count and sedimentation rate
   3. May have aseptic meningitis, arthralgia, arthritis, proteinemia, sterile pyuria, diarrhea, abnormal liver function tests
C. Diagnosis
   Clinical signs and symptoms
D. Complications
   1. Myocardial infarction (can be fatal)
   2. Coronary aneurysm

E. Treatment
   1. Aspirin
   2. Symptomatic
   3. Monitor ECG and echocardiogram

JUVENILE RHEUMATOID ARTHRITIS
(STILL'S DISEASE) (Fig. 97)

A. Definition
   Systemic disease involving joints, connective tissue, viscera
B. Epidemiology and Etiology
   1. Onset rare before 6 months of age
   2. More common in girls
   3. Etiology unknown but infection and immune disorder have received most attention
   4. Emotional stress linked to onset and exacerbation
   5. Age of onset
     a. Can occur any time during pediatric period
     b. Peak incidence below 5-year and in 10- to 15-year age groups
   6. Family history
     Increased incidence of rheumatoid arthritis and history of juvenile rheumatoid arthritis
C. Manifestations
   1. Monoarticular-polyarticular disease
     a. Splenomegaly or hepatomegaly not present
     b. Little or no lymphadenopathy
   2. Still's disease (Still's triad)
     a. Polyarthritis
     b. Hepatosplenomegaly
     c. Lymphadenopathy
   3. Acute onset disease
     a. Splenomegaly or hepatomegaly not present
     b. Lymphadenopathy
     c. Mild arthritis and/or arthralgia
     d. Rash
     e. Fever
   4. Fever
     Patterns of fever
       1. Intermittent daily high spike with return to normal or near normal (in Still's type)
       2. Periods of normal temperature followed by low-grade and intermediate fever spikes

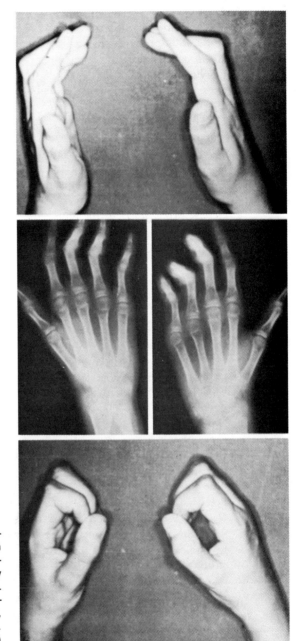

Fig. 97. Juvenile rheumatoid arthritis. Dry arthritis in a child with painless, general systemic polyarthritis. Mobility is severely limited by loss of extra-articular tissue stretch. Note the lack of swelling and well-maintained joint space. (*Boone JE, et al: Juvenile rheumatoid arthritis. Pediatr Clin North Am 21:885, 1974*)

3. Low-grade fever with mild elevation in late afternoon or evening (monoarticular-polyarticular type)
5. Morning stiffness
6. Rash
   a. Erythematous, pink, circumscribed, macular or maculopapular lesions on trunk, ventral side or arms, medial aspects of thighs, buttocks, face
   b. Usually precipitated by fever or warm bath
   c. Usually nonpruritic
7. Subcutaneous nodules
   a. Occur in about 10% of cases
   b. On hands, elbows, shins
   c. Associated with severe relapses
8. Splenomegaly
   a. Occurs primarily in Still's type
   b. Spleen is firm, nontender
   c. Enlargement can be massive
9. Lympadenopathy
   a. Usually generalized
   b. Occurs in Still's type
   c. Lymph nodes usually nontender, firm, smooth, well circumscribed
10. Ocular involvement
    a. Occurs in about 10% of patients
    b. Can involve iris, ciliary body, lens, cornea (scleral, choroid involvement rare)
    c. Usually presents insidiously as iritis (asymmetry of pupils) with later involvement of ciliary body (iridocyclitis)
    d. If untreated, cornea becomes involved and cataracts and band keratopathy can develop
    e. Lesions usually bilateral and frequently occur months or years after initial arthritic symptoms
11. Cardiac involvement
    a. Potentially lethal but usually has benign course
    b. Usually pericarditis and/or myocarditis (Fig. 98)
    c. Seen most often with acute onset disease
    d. An indication for steroid therapy
12. Vasculitis
    a. Vasculitis uncommon
    b. Skin manifestations include petecheae and ecchymoses or erythematous, tender, indurated areas
13. Renal involvement
    Low incidence
14. Joint involvement
    a. Manifested by pain, heat, swelling, mild erythema
    b. Small joints affected in particular

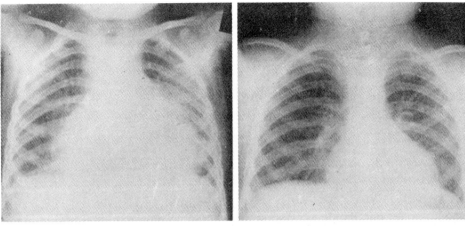

Fig. 98. Juvenile rheumatoid arthritis. Pericarditis is an indication for aggressive steroid treatment. One can expect a dramatic response, like the one that occurred here, in 7 days. (*Boone JE et al: Juvenile rheumatoid arthritis. Pediatr Clin North Am 21:885, 1974*)

    15. Laboratory and serologic tests
        a. Hemogram shows elevated leukocyte count, elevated erythrocyte sedimentation rate, anemia
        b. Rheumatoid factor test not particularly helpful
D. Diagnosis
    1. Clinical signs and symptoms
        a. Polyarticular changes
        b. Chronic course (3 months or more)
        c. Exclusion of other chronic joint disorders
        d. Onset of symptoms before age 15 years
    2. Hemogram
E. Treatment
    Acute disease
    a. Salicylates
    b. Ibuprofen (if salicylate intolerance develops)
    c. Indomethacin (if salicylates ineffective)
    d. Corticosteroids (if other therapy ineffective)
    e. Physical therapy

SYSTEMIC LUPUS ERYTHEMATOSUS (SLE)
(Fig. 99)

A. Definition
    A potentially fatal chronic collagen disease of variable severity with widespread involvement

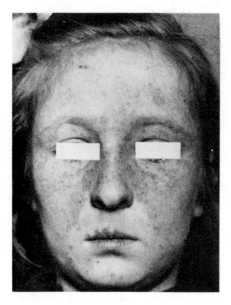

Fig. 99. Typical "butterfly" rash of disseminated lupus erythematosus. (*Hutchison JH: Practical Paediatric Problems, p 596. Lloyd-Luke Publication. Chicago, Year Book (distributor) 1975*)

B. Etiology
　　1. Unknown
　　2. A lupuslike illness may be induced by variety of drugs including **hydralazine,** anticonvulsants, procainamide, isoniazid
　　　　a. Usually mild and reversible if **offending agent is withdrawn**
C. Clinical features
　　1. Widespread involvement of multiple organs
　　2. Usually in girls over 8 years of age
　　3. Onset insidious or acute
　　4. Raynaud's phenomenon* may be present
　　5. Alopecia may occur
　　6. Erythema nodosum
　　7. Erythema multiforme
　　8. Thrombocytopenia with purpura
　　9. Arthralgia or arthritis common
　　10. Myositis, muscle weakness, pain
　　11. Aseptic necrosis of femoral head
　　12. Hepatosplenomegaly and generalized lymphadenopathy
　　13. Polyserositis (pleuritis, pericarditis, peritonitis) common
　　14. Myocarditis
　　15. Endocarditis (Libman-Sacks disease)
　　16. Neurologic symptoms (peripheral neuritis, **central nervous system disease,** psychiatric disturbance)

* See Glossary

17. Anemia, leukopenia
18. Renal involvement in most children
D. Diagnosis and Laboratory Findings
    Diagnosis based on typical multisystem disease and confirmed by laboratory tests
    a. Antinuclear antibody test almost always positive (but not necessarily diagnostic)
    b. Also, elevated immunoglobulins, positive serologic test for syphilis commonly present
    c. Anemia, thrombocytopenia, leukopenia may be present
    d. Liver function tests may be abnormal
    e. Hematuria, pyuria, red cell casts, proteinurea, and sometimes classic findings of nephrotic syndrome
    f. Low serum complement levels
    g. Renal biopsy shows characteristic histologic picture
E. Treatment
    1. Symptomatic, antimalarials, low-dose corticosteroid therapy for mild disease without nephritis
    2. Large doses of corticosteroids for prolonged periods of time for severe disease
F. Complications and Prognosis
    1. Prognosis related to severity of disease
    2. Nephritis, central nervous system disease, infection are most common causes of death
    3. Other causes of death include myocardial infarction, malignancy, pulmonary SLE, suicide
    4. Early recognition and vigorous therapy has resulted in 90% survival rate beyond 5 years

RHEUMATIC FEVER

A. Definition
    A poststreptococcal disease characterized by nonsuppurative inflammation, particularly the heart
B. Etiologic Considerations and Pathogenesis
    1. Is the most common cause of acquired heart disease in children and adolescents
    2. Frequency and severity decreasing in United States in recent decades
    3. Is a sequela of group A streptococcal infections of upper respiratory tract (latent period is 1–5 weeks)
    4. Attack rate after untreated group A streptococcal upper respiratory infection is about 3% but may be related to severity of infection
    5. Does not follow group A streptococcal pyoderma, as may acute glomerulonephritis
    6. Attacks rare under 3 years of age

      7. Disease is more frequent, more severe, and occurs at an earlier age in underdeveloped countries

C. Clinical Features

  1. Carditis

    a. Endocardium, myocardium, pericardium may be involved

    b. Incidence of carditis 40–50% following initial attack of rheumatic fever

    c. Becomes manifest during first 2 weeks of disease

    d. Signs of carditis include cardiac murmurs, pericardial friction rub, cardiomegaly, congestive heart failure

    e. Mitral valve most commonly involved with aortic valve being next in frequency (mitral insufficiency, mitral stenosis, aortic insufficiency, aortic stenosis)

  2. Arthritis

    a. In about 25% of patients

    b. Usually is chief complaint

    c. *Large* joints involved (one or more)

    d. Affected joints are red, hot, swollen, painful

    e. May involve several joints simultaneously or may migrate from joint to joint

    f. Clears without permanent joint damage

    g. Some have arthralgia rather than arthritis

  3. Sydenham's chorea

    a. Appears after a longer latent period (2–6 months)

    b. May be initial complaint

    c. Characterized by purposeless motions, poor neuromuscular control, emotional lability

    d. May have associated carditis

    e. More frequent in girls

    f. Duration weeks to months

  4. Erythema marginatum

    a. In about 10% of patients

    b. Faint red macules that enlarge and clear in center leaving ringlike lesions

    c. On trunk and proximal extremities

    d. Arthritis and carditis frequently associated

  5. Subcutaneous nodules

    a. In less than 10% of patients

    b. Small nodules over pressure points (elbows, knees, scalp)

  6. Other less specific manifestations

    a. Fever and malaise

    b. Abdominal pain

    c. Epistaxis

    d. Rheumatic pneumonitis (rare)

    e. Hematuria (rare)

    f. Electrocardiographic abnormalities (prolonged P-R interval), gallop rhythm, tachycardia

TABLE 3 Jones Criteria for Diagnosis of Rheumatic Fever

MAJOR CRITERIA	MINOR CRITERIA	SUPPORTIVE EVIDENCE

Carditis
Polyarthritis
Chorea
Erythema marginatum
Subcutaneous nodules
	History of previous rheumatic
	  fever
	Arthralgia
	Fever
	Increased erythrocyte sedimenta-
	  tion rate, anemia, leukocytosis,
	  positive C-reactive protein
	Prolonged P-R interval on electro-
	  cardiogram
		Recent streptococcal upper respi-
		  ratory infection
		Throat culture positive for group
		  A streptococci
		Increased antistreptolysin (ASO)
		  titer or other streptococcal anti-
		  bodies

D. Diagnosis and Laboratory Findings
1. Is a clinical diagnosis; it should not be made lightly
2. Based on Jones criteria (Table 3): 2 major or 1 major and 2 minor criteria with evidence of recent streptococcal infection suggest high probability of rheumatic fever
3. "Pure chorea" patients may not have laboratory evidence of preceding streptococcal infection because of long latent period

E. Treatment
1. When first seen, should be treated with penicillin (to eradicate streptococci), and penicillin prophylaxis against further streptococcal infection should be instituted (incidence of recurrent rheumatic fever with subsequent streptococcal infections is 20–50%)
2. Salicylates alone if no carditis
3. Salicylates and corticosteroids if carditis is present
4. Indications and use of corticosteroids still somewhat controversial
5. Bed rest (controversial)
6. Therapy for chorea is purely supportive

BIBLIOGRAPHY

Grossman BJ, Mukhopadhyay D: Juvenile rheumatoid arthritis. Curr Probl Pediatr 5:3–61, 1975

Kegel SM et al: Cardiac death in mucocutaneous lymph node syndrome. Am J Cardiol 40:282–286, 1977

Mucocutaneous lymph node syndrome. Morbidity and Mortality Weekly Report 27:9, 1978

Stiehm ER, Fulginiti VA: Immunologic Disorders in Infants and Children. Philadelphia, W. B. Saunders, 1980

18

Neuromuscular Disorders

PSEUDOHYPERTROPHIC MUSCULAR DYSTROPHY

A. General Considerations
  1. Commonest form is *childhood* or Duchenne type
  2. Usually sex-linked inherited disease classically in boys
B. Manifestations
  1. Usually not recognized until age 2–3 years
  2. Late onset of sitting, walking, running
  3. Waddling gait
  4. Difficulty in climbing stairs
  5. Hypertrophy of calf muscles
  6. Lordosis
  7. Gower's sign (rises from floor by assuming prone position, kneeling, then raising self to standing by pushing hands against shins, knees, and thighs, Fig. 100)
  8. Profound muscle atrophy in late stages
  9. Progressive deterioration with death usually before 20 years

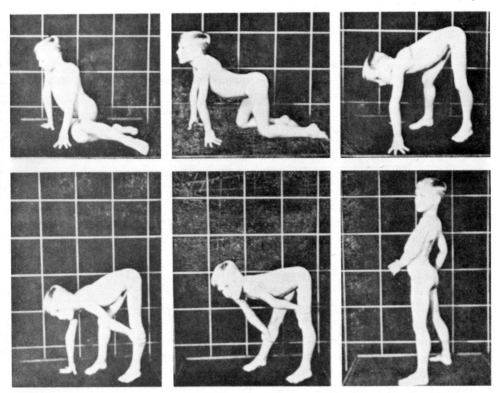

Fig. 100. A child 7 years of age with pseudohypertrophic muscular dystrophy, showing characteristic manner of rising from the floor. The last picture shows the standing position with severe lordosis. (*Huttenlocher PR: In Vaughan VC III, McKay RJ, Nelson WE (eds): Nelson Textbook of Pediatrics, p 1468. Philadelphia, W. B. Saunders, 1975*)

    10. Cardiac muscle also involved and cardiomyopathy may occasionally be cause of death

C. Diagnosis

    Confirmed by electromyography, muscle biopsy, and elevated serum enzymes (particularly CPK but also SGOT and aldolase)

D. Treatment

    1. No effective treatment

    2. Orthopaedic consultation

    3. Genetic counseling

FLOPPY CHILD SYNDROME

General Considerations

1. Includes a heterogeneous group of infants with weak, hypotonic muscles and varying degrees of flaccid paralysis

2. Symptoms may appear at birth or later in infancy
3. Prognosis is variable depending on underlying disease
4. Progression may be slow or rapid and terminate in death. Process may become arrested with partial or complete recovery
5. May be due to diseases of cerebrum, cerebellum, spinal cord peripheral nerves, neuromuscular junctions, or muscle
6. Most common cause is degeneration or malformation of spinal cord anterior horn cells (*Werdnig-Hoffman disease,* Fig. 101)
   a. Absent tendon reflexes
   b. Fibrillations of tongue usually visible
   c. Onset before 2 years of age
   d. Death results from respiratory failure
7. *Benign congenital hypotonia* may be difficult to distinguish from Werdnig-Hoffman disease early in its course but eventual recovery clearly establishes diagnosis

INFANT BOTULISM

A. General Considerations
   1. First recognized in 1976
   2. 15 cases reported in 1976 and 42 cases in 1977
   3. Seems to be widespread throughout United States
B. Etiology
   1. Due to ingestion of *Clostridium botulinum* spores found generally in soil. Spores develop in infantile gut and produce toxin. Gut of older children and adults not conducive to this
   2. Honey implicated as one source of infection
C. Manifestations
   1. Abrupt onset in previously well infant
   2. Age at onset 3–26 weeks
   3. Constipation, lethargy, difficulty in feeding and swallowing, generalized weakness, hypotonia, weak cry, respiratory distress, pooling of oral secretions, ptosis, pneumonia
   4. Neuromuscular paralysis
D. Treatment
   1. Hospitalization
   2. Supportive therapy including assisted ventilation
   3. Death may result from respiratory arrest
   4. Aminoglycosides accentuate symptoms and are thus contraindicated

MYASTHENIA GRAVIS

A. General Considerations
   1. Characterized by weakness and fatigue of voluntary muscles with tendency to recover after rest. Symptoms more pronounced in afternoon and evenings

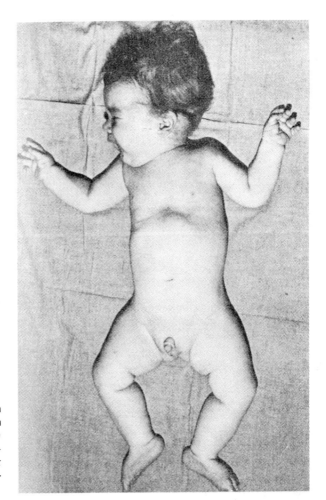

Fig. 101. Typical posture of an infant with Werdnig-Hoffmann disease. (*Huttenlocher PR: In Vaughan VC III, McKay RJ, Nelson WE (eds): Nelson Textbook of Pediatrics, p 1459. Philadelphia, W. B. Saunders, 1975*)

2. Ocular movements, facial expression, mastication, deglutition, and speech are affected primarily, but neck, trunk, and limbs may also be involved
3. Respiratory embarrassment occurs in severe cases
4. May develop at any age
5. Three forms in infancy and childhood
    a. *Neonatal transient form:* Occurs in some infants born of mothers with disease. Symptoms include hypotonia, poor cry and suck, impaired breathing and swallowing. Diagnosis established by response to edrophonium chloride (Tensilon). With continued therapy, complete recovery occurs within 2 months
    b. *Congenital myasthenia gravis:* Occurs in infants born of unaffected mothers. In contrast to transient neonatal type, involvement of bulbar musculature is rare. Complete remission of disease is rare

   c. *Juvenile myasthenia gravis:* Onset usually after 10 years of age. Primary lesion involves defective transmission of impulses at neuromuscular junction

B. Treatment
1. Anticholinesterase drugs [pyridostigmine bromide (Mestinon), neostigmine (Prostigmin), ambenonium chloride (Mytelase)]
2. Thymectomy of particular value in young females

C. Course and Prognosis

Prolonged and characterized by remissions and relapses. With therapy, remission may be complete and may last for up to 6 years. Most children can lead near normal lives with optimum therapy

BIBLIOGRAPHY

Follow-up on infant botulism—United States. Morbidity and Mortality Weekly Report 27:17–18, 23, 1978

Hoekelman RA et al: Principles of Pediatrics, Health Care of the Young. New York, McGraw-Hill, 1978

Honey exposure and infant botulism. Morbidity and Mortality Weekly Report 27:249–255, 1978

Merten DF et al: Infant botulism and constipation. Roentgenol 131:523–524, 1978

McKee KT Jr et al: Another case of botulism in infancy. Am J Dis Child 131:857–859, 1977

Polin RA, Brown LW: Infant botulism. Pediatr Clin North Am 26:345–354, 1979

Rudolph AM, Barnett HL, Einhorn AH: Pediatrics. New York, Appleton-Century-Crofts, 1977

Vaughan VC III, McKay RJ, Nelson WE: Nelson Textbook of Pediatrics. Philadelphia, W. B. Saunders, 1975

19

Ocular Disorders

STRABISMUS

A. General Considerations
1. Affects about 3% of children
2. Definition

   Deviation of one eye due to imbalance of extraocular muscles (cross-eye, squint)
3. Types of strabismus
   a. *Phoria:* Eyes are perfectly aligned except when fusion is prevented (*i.e.*, closing one eye, fatigue)
   b. *Tropia:* A persistent deviation that cannot be corrected by effort
   c. *Esotropia and esophoria:* Eye deviates inwardly
   d. *Exotropia and exophoria:* Eye deviates outwardly
   e. *Alternating strabismus:* Either eye may be used for fixation while other eye deviates

B. Esotropia
1. May be congenital or acquired

2. Congenital type not influenced by medical treatment. Requires surgical correction
3. Acquired type often a result of hyperopia (farsightedness)
   a. Onset usually 1–4 years of age
   b. Suitable glasses and miotics in early years often result in permanent correction of strabismus
   c. Surgery not indicated if due to hyperopia
C. Exotropia
   1. Initially intermittent (exophoria)
   2. Early onset, often shortly after birth
   3. Little or no refractive error
   4. Becomes exaggerated when focusing on distant objects or with tiring
   5. With time, affected eye may become suppressed and lead to constant deviation (exotropia)
   6. Treatment consists of orthoptics* or surgery
   7. Exotropia almost always a surgical problem
D. Diagnosis
   1. In tropias, clinical appearance of persistent eye deviation
   2. In phorias, history of intermittent eye deviation, cover test* and cover–uncover test*
E. Complications
   1. Amblyopia (permanent impairment of vision resulting from disuse of deviating eye)
   2. Ocular torticollis (tilting of head in an effort to achieve binocular single vision)

NYSTAGMUS

A. Definition
   Rhythmic involuntary oscillations of one or both eyes (usually both) in any of the directions of gaze
B. General Considerations
   1. May be *pendular* (to-and-fro motions of equal speed) or *jerk nystagmus* (slow component in one direction and rapid in other)
   2. Direction may be horizontal, vertical, rotatory, mixed
   3. Amplitude is fine, medium, or coarse
C. Etiology and Significance
   1. Physiologic types
      a. *Optokinetic nystagmus:* Occurs normally under conditions such as watching scenery from moving vehicle. Is a jerk nystagmus of no pathologic significance
      b. *Evoked vestibular nystagmus:* Dependent on impulses from semicircular

* See Glossary

canals and occurs for example with irrigation of ear canal. Is a jerk nystagmus of no pathologic significance
- c. *End-position nystagmus:* Occurs with extreme lateral gaze. Is a jerk nystagmus of no pathologic significance
- d. *Voluntary nystagmus:* A pendular nystagmus that can be induced by will. Of no pathologic significance
2. Pathologic types
- a. "Ocular" or "neurologic" nystagmus due to defects in eye or lesions in posterior fossa or motor pathways. Ocular tends to be perpendicular; neurologic may be either pendular or jerky
- b. *Hereditary pendular nystagmus* is of ocular type, may lessen with age but persists throughout life
- c. *Spasmus nutans* consists of pendular nystagmus (ocular), head nodding, torticollis. Etiology obscure. Onset during first year or two of life and persists for only a few months
- d. *Unilateral pendular nystagmus* (ocular) may develop with loss of vision in one eye
- e. *Congenital jerk nystagmus* (ocular) develops early and persists throughout life. Etiology unknown. Hereditary in some cases
- f. *Acquired fixational nystagmus* (neurologic), pendular or jerky, horizontal or vertical. An ominous sign of neurologic disease
- g. In addition to ocular and neurologic nystagmus, may have "vestibular" nystagmus. Latter is jerk nystagmus that may result from peripheral or central vestibular dysfunction

CATARACT (CONGENITAL OR INFANTILE)
(Fig. 102)

A. Definition

An opacity of crystalline lens
B. General Considerations
1. Congenital cataracts present at birth but often not discovered until later
2. Vary in size from small dot to clouding of entire lens
3. Congenital cataracts usually remain stationary but may progress
4. Congenital cataracts may be *partial* (nuclear, anterior, posterior, lamellar, zonular) or *complete*
C. Etiology
1. Many times cause cannot be determined
2. Congenital cataracts may be hereditary, familial, or associated with intrauterine infections (*i.e.*, rubella), inborn errors of metabolism (*i.e.*, galactosemia), intraocular disease (*i.e.*, congenital glaucoma), trauma, drugs (corticosteroids), chromosomal aberrations (trisomies), neurologic abnormalities

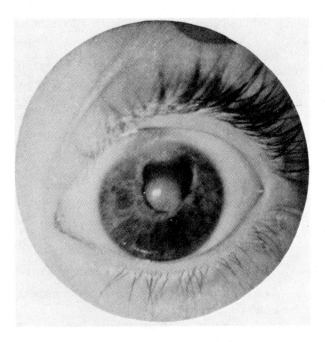

Fig. 102. Typical rubella cataract in microphthalmic eye following iridectomy. (*McDonald PR: In Harley RD (ed): Pediatric Ophthalmology, p 383. Philadelphia, W. B. Saunders, 1975*)

D. Treatment

  Patients should be referred to ophthalmologist early so that surgery can be considered

E. Visual Prognosis

  Guarded. Best in patients with bilateral partial cataracts. Patients with complete unilateral cataracts almost always develop severe amblyopia even after surgery

CONGENITAL GLAUCOMA (Fig. 103)

A. Definition

  Increased intraocular pressure appearing at or shortly after birth

B. General Considerations

  1. More common in males
  2. Transmitted as autosomal recessive
  3. Increase in pressure due to obstruction of aqueous humor flow as a result of developmental anomalies of angle structures

C. Manifestations

  1. Extreme photophobia common
  2. Blepharospasm* and tearing usually associated
  3. Corneal haziness, edema and congestion of conjunctiva, increased diameter of

  * See Glossary

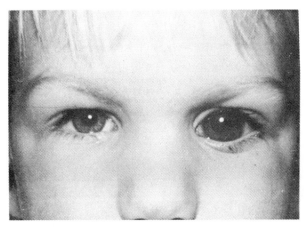

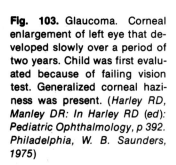

Fig. 103. Glaucoma. Corneal enlargement of left eye that developed slowly over a period of two years. Child was first evaluated because of failing vision test. Generalized corneal haziness was present. (*Harley RD, Manley DR: In Harley RD (ed): Pediatric Ophthalmology, p 392. Philadelphia, W. B. Saunders, 1975*)

cornea, increased intraocular pressure, enlargement of globe, linear opacities in cornea, optic nerve atrophy

D. Diagnosis
   1. Manifestations
   2. Measurement of intraocular pressure under anesthesia (normal pressure usually not over 18 mm Hg)
   3. Must be differentiated from secondary glaucoma associated with a host of other causes such as rubella syndrome, Lowe's syndrome, Sturge-Weber syndrome
E. Treatment
   Early surgery essential
F. Prognosis
   1. The earlier the onset, the worse the prognosis
   2. Long-term visual results not good even if intraocular pressure is restored to normal

BLEPHARITIS

General Considerations
1. A common chronic, recurrent inflammation of margins of lids. Characterized by scaling, redness, loss of lashes
2. *Staphylococcic blepharitis* often associated with ulcers or tiny pustules
3. *Seborrheic blepharitis* (*squamous blepharatis*) characterized by greasy scales. Seborrhea of scalp and brows commonly associated
   May be complicated by staphylococcal infection
4. Treatment consists of antibiotic ointments (bacitracin, tetracycline, sulfacetamide) for staphylococcal type, corticosteroid ointment for seborrheic type, and combination of both for mixed type

HORDEOLUM (STY)

General Considerations
1. Infection (usually staphylococcal) of ciliary follicle beginning as circumscribed tender swelling progressing to suppuration and rupture
2. Treatment consists of intermittent warm, moist compresses (not more than 20 minutes at any one time) and application of antistaphylococcal ointment

CHALAZIAN

General Considerations
1. A slow-growing firm round mass in the tarsus* of the eyelid due to retention of secretions of a meibomian gland
2. Not accompanied by pain or tenderness
3. May resorb spontaneously
4. May require incision and drainage by ophthalmologist

CONJUNCTIVITIS

General Considerations
1. Inflammation of bulbar and lacrimal conjunctiva associated with redness, swelling, and tearing or exudate depending on cause
2. Due to wide variety of causes including chemical irritation (*i.e.*, silver nitrate instillation in newborn), bacterial infection (*i.e.*, *N. gonorrhea*), viral infection (*i.e.*, *Chlamydia trachomatis*), allergies
3. Treatment depends on cause. Instillation of antibiotic ointments for infectious types. Corticosteroid ointments may be useful for allergic conjunctivitis

IRITIS

General Considerations
1. Inflammation of the iris
2. Characterized by pain, photophobia, contraction of pupil, and discoloration of iris, but symptoms may be minimal
3. Patient must be referred to ophthalmologist because permanent ocular damage and blindness may result

* See Glossary

FOREIGN BODIES

General Considerations
1. *Conjunctival foreign bodies* can generally be easily removed with cotton-tipped applicator. If foreign body not visible, upper eyelid should be everted and inspected
2. *Corneal foreign bodies* are potentially more serious. May require instillation of fluorescein to demonstrate presence. If foreign body cannot be removed with cotton-tipped applicator, patient should be referred to ophthalmologist

CORNEAL ABRASIONS

General Considerations
1. Associated with marked blephoraspasm, tearing, pain
2. Treatment consists of initial instillation of topical anesthetic to relieve pain and permit satisfactory examination (topical anesthesia not to be used chronically). Antibiotic ointment and eye patch
3. Usually heal promptly but should be followed closely for signs of infection

RETINOBLASTOMA

A. General Considerations
   1. Most common intraocular tumor in infants and children
   2. Is a congenital malignant tumor consisting of embryonal retinal cells
   3. Always congenital but may not be discovered until late infancy or early childhood
   4. Involvement is bilateral in 30% of cases
   5. Familial occurrence associated with autosomal dominant transmission
B. Manifestations
   1. Initial sign may be only strabismus secondary to visual impairment. For this reason, *every young pediatric patient with strabismus requires thorough ophthalmoscopic examination*
   2. With growth, creamy white pupillary reflex is seen ("cat's eye") and tumor mass can be easily visualized
   3. Abnormality often first noted by parents
C. Course
   May spread locally or invade optic nerve and extend to brain, causing death. Bone metastases rare
D. Treatment and Prognosis
   1. If unilateral and small, prompt enucleation results in 90% chance of survival
   2. If optic nerve is involved, cure rate reduced to 50%
   3. Extension to cranium or orbit carries poor prognosis

4. If bilateral, more involved eye is enucleated and remaining eye treated with radiation and chemotherapy. If involvement is extensive in both eyes, then bilateral enucleation is indicated
5. Spontaneous regression rare

BIBLIOGRAPHY

Harley RD: Pediatric Ophthalmology. Philadelphia, W. B. Saunders, 1976.

Hoekelman RA et al: Principles of Pediatrics. Health Care of the Young. New York, McGraw-Hill, 1978

Rudolph AM, Barnett HL, Einhorn AH: Pediatrics. New York, Appleton-Century-Crofts, 1977

Vaughan VC III, McKay RJ, Nelson WE: Nelson Textbook of Pediatrics. Philadelphia, W. B. Saunders, 1975

20 | Nasal Disorders

TRAUMA

General Considerations
1. Common cause of epistaxis
2. May result in fracture of bony and cartilaginous structures with resultant deformity. Fractures may involve sinuses, orbit, anterior cranial fossa. Crystal clear rhinorrhea with high glucose content indicates extension into anterior cranial fossa with leakage of cerebrospinal fluid
3. Simple fractures without displacement require no treatment

FOREIGN BODIES

General Considerations
1. More common in infants and mentally retarded children
2. Unilateral foul-smelling discharge is due to foreign body until proved otherwise
3. Removal may have to be accomplished under general anesthesia

EPISTAXIS

General Considerations
1. Usually due to trauma, allergic rhinitis, chronic infection
2. May be a manifestation of blood dyscrasia
3. Generally ceases with occlusion of nares, mouth breathing, reassurance
4. Severe cases may require nasal packs
5. Chronic recurrent epistaxis due to localized ulceration may require cauterization

MOUTH BREATHING

General Considerations
1. During early months of life, infants are obligate nose breathers, and obstruction of nares causes respiratory difficulty
2. In early childhood, adenoid obstruction is common cause
3. At any age beyond period of infancy, allergic rhinitis is common cause
4. Acute mouth breathing usually due to upper respiratory infection
5. Chronic mouth breathing causes "pinched" appearance of face ("adenoid facies")
6. Treatment consists of identification and correction of cause

CHOANAL ATRESIA

General Considerations
1. Atresia of nasal choanae is rare congenital abnormality
2. Generally recognized shortly after birth
3. Diagnosis suspected by respiratory distress and confirmed by inability to pass nasal catheter. Also confirmed by roentgenogram after instillation of radiopaque substance
4. If bilateral, tracheotomy may be required
5. Surgery eventually required. If infant can compensate for nasal obstruction and tolerate condition, surgery best delayed for 6–12 months

NASAL POLYPOSIS

General Considerations
1. Occurs primarily with allergic rhinitis and cystic fibrosis
2. Polyps are chronic pedunculated masses of edematous nasal mucosa
3. Cause chronic nasal obstruction, nasal discharge
4. May be single or multiple, appear as whitish avascular shiny masses
5. If removed, tend to recur unless basis is identified and corrected

DEVIATION OF NASAL SEPTUM

General Considerations
1. Rare in young children
2. Usually acquired secondary to trauma
3. Surgery only rarely required
4. If surgery is indicated, it is best not performed before puberty or external deformity of nose may result

PERFORATION OF NASAL SEPTUM

General Considerations
1. A rare condition
2. May be congenital, frequently associated with cleft lip and cleft palate
3. Usually caused by syphilis, tuberculosis, trauma

BIBLIOGRAPHY

Hoekelman RA et al: Principles of Pediatrics. Health Care of the Young. New York, McGraw-Hill, 1978

Rudolph AM, Barnett HL, Einhorn AH: Pediatrics. New York, Appleton-Century-Crofts, 1977

Vaughan VC III, McKay RJ, Nelson WE: Nelson Textbook of Pediatrics. Philadelphia, W. B. Saunders, 1975

21

Chromosomal Disorders

DOWN'S SYNDROME (MONGOLISM, TRISOMY 21)
(Fig. 104)

A. General Considerations
    1. Incidence about 1–5 per 1000 births
    2. May occur with any maternal age but more common if mother is over 35 years or father is over 55 years
    3. Majority of patients have 47 chromosomes with trisomy of chromosome 21
    4. Small percentage have 46 chromosomes with translocation. This type seen with younger mothers
    5. Etiology unknown
B. Manifestations
    1. Trisomy 21 and translocation clinically indistinguishable
    2. Clinical features
        a. Microcephaly, brachycephaly*
        b. Brushfield's spots (speckling of iris bilaterally)

* See Glossary

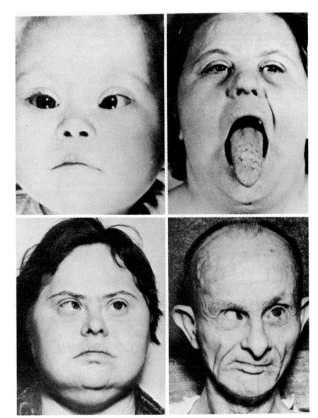

Fig. 104. Facies of four patients of varying ages with Down's syndrome. Note flattening of the nasal bridge, orbital ridges and maxillae, fissuring of the tongue, oblique palpebral fissures, epicanthal folds, spotting of the iris, and strabismus. It is important to note that as these patients age their facial features become altered. (*Goodman RM, Gorlin RJ: The Face in Genetic Disorders, p 59. Saint Louis, C. V. Mosby, 1970*)

   c. Strabismus

   d. Low-set ears

   e. Large fissured tongue

   f. Small nasopharynx

   g. Mouth breathing

   h. Abnormal or missing teeth

   i. Short, thick neck

   j. Stubby hands, short inwardly curved fifth finger (clinodactyly), single mid-palmar crease (simian line)

   k. Wide space between first and second toes

   l. Umbilical hernia

  m. Dry skin

   n. Hypotonia

   o. Congenital heart disease (more commonly endocardial cushion defect or ventricular septal defect)

   p. Undescended testes, small penis

   q. Roentgenogram of pelvis shows wide iliac wings

    r. Absence of breast tissue is helpful clue in neonatal period

    s. Upward slant of palpebral fissures

  3. Intelligence

       Intelligence level variable but all are retarded

  4. Development

    a. All aspects of development are retarded

    b. Aging process is rapid (cataracts not uncommon in adult life)

C. Associated Disorders

  1. Duodenal atresia

  2. Megacolon

  3. Leukemia

  4. Malfunction of thyroid, pituitary, adrenal glands

  5. Intercurrent respiratory infections

D. Diagnosis

  1. Clinical features

  2. Confirmed by chromosome analysis

E. Genetic Counseling

  1. All children with Down's syndrome should have chromosome studies

  2. If infant has trisomy 21 and karyotype of mother is normal, risk of trisomy 21 in subsequent pregnancies is low but *only if mother is under 35 years of age*

  3. If infant has translocation or mosaicism, chromosome studies should be carried out on both parents and siblings to detect phenotypic carriers

F. Treatment

  1. Development is enhanced with tender loving care and retention of baby in home

  2. In selected cases, placement outside the home may be necessary depending on circumstances and feelings of family

TRISOMY 13 SYNDROME (D TRISOMY) (Fig. 105)

A. General Considerations

  1. Incidence 1 in 4000–5000 births

  2. Syndrome associated with an additional chromosome (No. 13) in the D group

  3. Older maternal age is a factor

  4. Infants generally small for gestational age

B. Manifestations

  1. Any organ system may be involved

  2. More common anomalies are cleft palate, cleft lip, microphthalmia,* hyperconvex narrow finger nails, midline defects, cryptorchidism, abnormal auricles, polydactyly, flexion of fingers, prominent heels, cardiac defects

  3. Cleft lip, cleft palate, microphthalmia with colobomata* are most common findings

  4. Cleft lip and palate may be severe with absence of nasal septum and philtrum

  5. A hooklike nucleus occurs in majority of polymorphonuclear leukocytes

* See Glossary

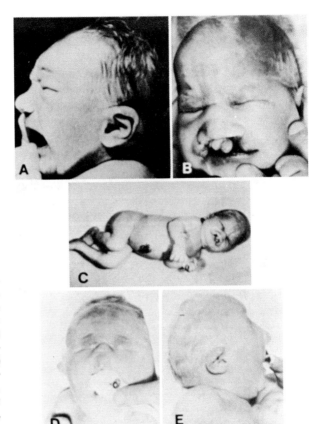

Fig. 105. Trisomy 13-15 syndrome. **(A-C)** Three infants who have various facial abnormalities including microcephaly, low-set and malformed ears, hairlip, capillary hemangioma, and small eyes. **(D)** Anophthalmia and a single external nares. (*Goodman RM, Gorling RJ: The Face in Genetic Disorders, p 155. Saint Louis, C. V. Mosby, 1970*)

6. Fetal hemoglobin persists in greater amounts than expected for age

C. Diagnosis
   1. Manifestations
   2. Chromosome studies show a whole extra 13 chromosome or an occasional mosaicism

D. Prognosis and Treatment
   1. Approximately 70% die within 3 months
   2. Correction of abnormalities generally not warranted
   3. Family support necessary
   4. Genetic counseling indicated

TRISOMY 18 SYNDROME (Fig. 106)

A. General Considerations
   1. Incidence 1 in about 3000 births
   2. Infants generally small for gestational age
   3. Associated with an additional 18 chromosome

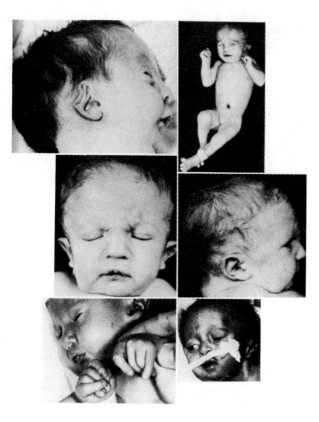

Fig. 106. Trisomy 18 syndrome. Infants who exhibit anteroposterior elongation of skull, micrognathia, hypertelorism, low-set and malformed ears, and short neck. In addition, one can note overlapped fingers, dorsiflexed big toe, and shield chest. (*Astley R: Br J Radiol 39: 86, 1966*)

    4. Older maternal age a factor

B. Manifestations

    1. Any organ system may be involved

    2. Most frequent defects are growth deficiency, developmental deficiency, malformed ears, micrognathia, flexed fingers with overlapping, short sternum, small pelvis, cryptorchidism, congenital heart disease

    3. Less common defects include simian crease, rocker-bottom feet, syndactyly of second and third toes

C. Diagnosis

    1. Clinical manifestations

    2. Chromosome studies usually show 47 chromosomes with a whole extra 18 chromosome. Occasional patient may be a mosaic

D. Prognosis and treatment

    1. Affected infants fail to thrive

    2. 60–70% die before 3 months of age

    3. Family support necessary

    4. Genetic counseling indicated

TURNER'S SYNDROME
(GONADAL DYSGENESIS) (Fig. 107)

A. Definition
1. Disorder of phenotypic females characterized by short stature, sexual infantilism, and "streak" gonads
2. Chromosome studies show 45X chromosomes, although varients and mosaics do exist
3. Sex-chromatin-negative buccal smear confirms diagnosis of 45X

B. Manifestations
1. Short stature
2. Shield chest
3. Webbed neck
4. Lymphedema
5. Short fourth metacarpal
6. Hypoplastic nails
7. Pigmented nevi
8. Congenital heart disease (particularly coarctation of aorta)
9. Streak gonads
10. Systemic hypertension
11. Renal anomalies (particularly horseshoe kidneys)
12. Cubitus valgus*
13. Late hearing defects
14. Mental deficiency (uncommon)
15. Spontaneous menstruation rare

C. Treatment
1. Psychologic counseling
2. Anabolic steroids to increase linear growth
3. Estrogen therapy to initiate feminization

NOONAN'S SYNDROME

A. General Considerations
1. Previously considered "male Turner's syndrome" but now is considered to include phenotypic males and females with normal karyotype but resembling Turner's syndrome
2. Synonyms include *XX and XY Turner phenotype, pseudo-Turner's syndrome, Ulrich's syndrome*

B. Manifestations
1. Short stature
2. Peculiar facies
3. Webbed neck

* See Glossary

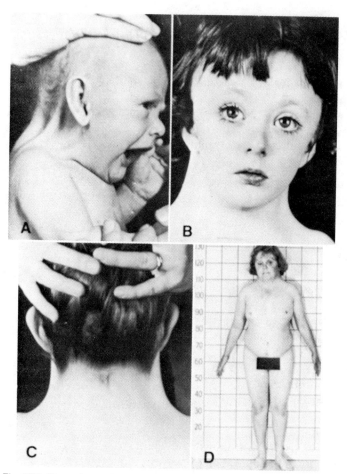

Fig. 107. Turner's syndrome. **(A–C)** Webbing of the neck, heart-shaped face, micrognathia, depressed corners of the mouth, and low hairline on the neck. **(D)** Short stature, shieldlike chest, widely spaced nipples with undeveloped breasts, surgical scar for repair of coarctation of the aorta, and cubitus valgus. *(Uchida AI et al: Am J Hum Genet 20:107, 1968; Hsu LYF et al: J Pediatr 79:12, 1971; Gustavson KH et al: Clin Genet 3:135, 1972)*

4 Congenital heart disease (most commonly pulmonic stenosis, atrial septal defect, or both)

5. Pectus excavatum, cubitus valgus, impaired mental development often present

6. Cryptorchidism and hypoplastic testes common in males

7. Females have functioning ovaries, and secondary sex characteristics appear but may be delayed

Fig. 108. Two untreated patients having Klinefelter's syndrome, who demonstrate the variations in Leydig cell function observed in this entity. **(A)** The small penis, decreased pubic hair, and sparse body hair indicate minimal androgen secretion. **(B)** Normal penile development and adequate pubic and body hair growth indicate essentially normal androgen production by the testis. Gynecomastia is also present. (*Paulsen CA: In Williams RH (ed): Textbook of Endocrinology, p 337. Philadelphia, W. B. Saunders, 1974*)

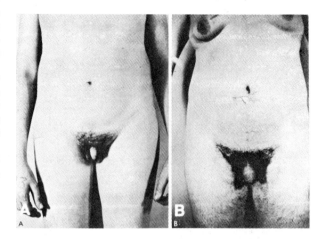

KLINEFELTER'S SYNDROME (Fig. 108)

A. General Considerations
   1. Is one of the most common forms of primary hypogonadism and infertility in males
   2. Hypogonadism and infertility caused by seminiferous tubule dysgenesis
   3. Have XXY sex chromosome constitution
   4. Less commonly, may have chromatin negative form (XY karyotype)
   5. Mosaicism has also been reported
   6. Incidence 1 in 500 males
B. Manifestations (chromatin-positive form)
   1. Small, firm testes only constant clinical feature
   2. Sterility
   3. Male phenotype
   4. Taller than average with relatively long legs
   5. Personality and behavioral disorders
   6. Intellectual subnormality
   7. Gynecomastia*
C. Associated Abnormalities
   1. Possible thyroid dysfunction
   2. Increased incidence of diabetes mellitus, usually mild
   3. Increased incidence of cancer of breast
   4. Possible increased incidence of chronic pulmonary disease and varicose veins

* See Glossary

BIBLIOGRAPHY

Gardner, LI: Endocrine and Genetic Diseases of Children and Adolescence. Philadelphia, W. B. Saunders, 1975

Hoekelman RA et al: Principles of Pediatrics. Health Care of the Young. New York, McGraw-Hill, 1978

McDonough PG: Gonadal dysgenesis and its variants. Pediatr Clin North Am 19:631–652, 1972

Rudolph AM, Barnett HL, Einhorn AH: Pediatrics. New York, Appleton-Century-Crofts, 1977

Vaughan VC III, McKay RJ, Nelson WE: Nelson Textbook of Pediatrics. Philadelphia, W. B. Saunders, 1975

Williams RH: Textbook of Endocrinology. Philadelphia, W. B. Saunders, 1974

22 | Orthopaedic Problems

FLATFOOT (PES PLANUS)

General Considerations
1. *Definition:* A low longitudinal arch
2. Low arch in infants is normal
3. Flatfoot *requires no treatment*
4. Pain or fatigue in feet, if present, *not* due to the low arch
5. Wearing sneakers does not cause or aggravate condition
6. Infants do not need shoes until they stand. Shoes should then be hard-soled

PIGEON TOE

General Considerations
1. Causes are *metatarsus varus, internal tibial torsion, internal femoral torsion*
2. *Metarsus varus*
   a. Consists of adduction of forefoot
   b. Hindfoot is normal

   c. Treatment must be instituted as soon as possible and definitely before infant walks

     1. Passive stretching by parent several times daily

     2. Reverse type shoes may be required

     3. In severe cases, orthopaedic consultation advised since casting may be necessary

  3. *Internal tibial torsion*

    Lower leg is twisted inwardly so that a line drawn from anterior superior iliac spine through center of patella (with foot in mid position) intersects fourth or fifth toe or beyond instead of second toe as normally

  4. *Internal femoral torsion*

    a. Same as internal tibial torsion except that upper leg is involved

    b. Diagnosis established by rotating hips inwardly and then patellae face each other—this is abnormal

    c. Requires no treatment when an isolated abnormality

EXTERNAL TIBIAL TORSION

General Considerations

1. Develops in most babies in neonatal period
2. By 2 years of age, almost all have some degree of external rotation
3. Does not require treatment when an isolated lesion

CLUBFOOT (Fig. 109)

A. General Considerations

  1. Types

    a. *Talipes equinovarus:* Inversion of heel and forefoot, adduction of forefoot, plantar flexion of entire foot

    b. *Talipes calcaneovalgus:* Eversion of heel and forefoot, abduction of forefoot, dorsiflexion of entire foot

  2. May be bilateral

  3. When present, neuromuscular and skeletal anomalies must be excluded

  4. Must be differentiated from functional deformities of newborn secondary to position *in utero*

    Functional deformities can be passively placed in neutral or even overcorrected position; anatomic clubfoot cannot

B. Treatment

  1. Early recognition crucial

  2. Orthopaedic consultation and early treatment (usually casting)

  3. In older children, surgical correction may be necessary

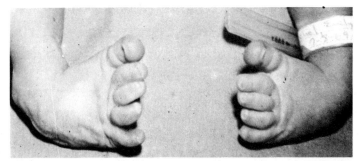

Fig. 109. Bilateral clubfoot in a child aged 2 weeks. (*Avery GB (ed): Neonatology. Philadelphia, JB Lippincott, 1975*)

PES CAVUS

General Considerations
1. Consists of unusually high longitudinal arch
2. Pathology is neuromuscular rather than bony
3. Generally does not appear until late childhood or adulthood
4. Is seen in association with neuromuscular diseases
5. Usually asymptomatic and requires no treatment
6. If severe, may require surgical correction

BOWLEGS (GENU VARUM)

General Considerations
1. When standing with ankles together, knees do not touch
2. Severe forms may occur with rickets
3. Usually requires no treatment
4. If severe, child should be carefully evaluated for underlying pathology and orthopaedic consultation sought

KNOCK-KNEES (GENU VALGUM)

General Considerations
1. When standing with knees together, ankles are apart
2. Severe forms may occur with rickets
3. Usually requires no treatment
4. If severe, child should be carefully evaluated for underlying pathology and orthopaedic consultation sought

CONGENITAL DISLOCATION OF HIP

A. General Considerations
   1. More accurately should be termed congenital dysplasia of hip. Head of femur may be partially or completely dislocated
   2. In United States, much more frequent in females
   3. Left side more commonly affected but can be bilateral
   4. Higher prevalence in cultures in which infants are swaddled (*i.e.,* American Indians)
   5. Less common in cultures in which infant is carried straddling mother's hip (*i.e.,* Orientals)
B. Diagnosis
   1. In neonatal period, subluxation may be recognized by deliberately manipulating femur into a dislocated position producing a "click" (Ortolani's maneuver).
   2. After 1–2 months, abduction of flexed hip becomes restricted (Fig. 110)
   3. Hips should be flexed and abducted on every office visit in early infancy. If knees do not nearly touch table, congenital dislocation of hip should be suspected
   4. With infant prone, gluteal folds not symmetric (often normal)
   5. X-ray examination of hips shows hip dysplasia with or without dislocation (Fig. 111)
C. Treatment
   1. Hips should be maintained in abduction
   2. In infants with positive Ortolani sign (subluxation but not dislocation), double diapering may be sufficient. If sign persists beyond a month or so or if limited hip abduction occurs, orthopaedic consultation should be requested
   3. If diagnosis is delayed beyond walking, operative procedures are necessary

TRANSIENT SYNOVITIS OF HIP JOINT

A. General Considerations
   1. Often referred to as "phantom hip"
   2. May be the earliest manifestation of Legg-Calvé-Perthes disease but is generally a self-limited nonspecific inflammatory process of hip
   3. Possible causes include viral diseases, remote infections, trauma
   4. More common in boys
B. Manifestations
   1. Painful hip and limp. Usually no pain with hip at rest
   2. May have history of recent upper respiratory infection
   3. Usually no history of trauma
   4. Pain usually present with *extremes of hip motion only* or while walking
   5. May have low-grade fever
   6. Roentgenogram usually normal but slight distention of joint space may be present

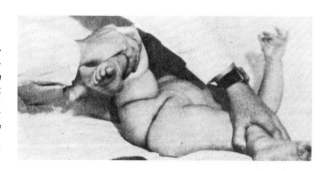

Fig. 110. Limitation of abduction is an early sign of congenital dislocation of the hip. Note restriction in abduction of right leg. (*Lachman JW: In Vaughan VC III, McKay RJ, Nelson WE (eds): Nelson Textbook of Pediatrics, p 1495. Philadelphia, W. B. Saunders, 1975*)

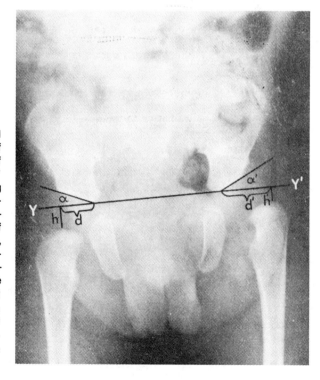

Fig. 111. Hilgenreiner's method for identification of dysplasia of the hip prior to ossification of the capital femoral epiphysis. α' is greater than α, indicating greater obliquity of the acetabular roof. d' is greater than d, indicating lateral displacement of the femur. h is greater than h', indicating cephalic displacement of the femur. These relations indicate dysplasia of the patient's left hip. (*Lachman JW: In Vaughan VC III, McKay RJ, Nelson WE (eds) Nelson Textbook of Pediatrics, p 1495. Philadelphia, W. B. Saunders, 1975*)

C. Diagnosis
   1. Aspiration not justified unless infection is suspected
   2. Manifestations usually sufficient to make correct diagnosis
D. Treatment
   1. Bed rest
   2. Symptoms usually disappear within 7–10 days
   3. Prolongation of symptoms or repeated recurrences should raise suspicion of Legg-Calvé-Perthes disease

LEGG-CALVÉ-PERTHES DISEASE (COXA PLANA)

A. General Considerations
   1. Is aseptic necrosis of head of femur with signs of synovitis
   2. Etiology unknown but may be due to an avascular process
   3. More common in boys
   4. Peak age prevalence 4–7 years
   5. May be complication of sickle cell disease or plaster hip spica in treatment of congenital dislocation of hip
   6. May be bilateral
B. Manifestations
   1. Begins as acute process that may be confused with transient synovitis of hip joint
   2. Painful hip *or knee* with flexion contracture of hip joint
   3. Symptoms relieved with rest
   4. Limp persists
C. Diagnosis
   1. X-ray examination shows flattening and fragmentation of femoral head with intact acetabulum
   2. Roentgenographic changes may be delayed for as long as a month after onset of symptoms
D. Treatment
   1. Should be referred to orthopaedist
   2. Treatment remains controversial. Some advocate long-term splinting, some advocate surgical repositioning
   3. If left untreated, condition will resolve spontaneously but with high incidence of secondary arthritis

THE OSTEOCHONDROSES

A. Definition
   Disease of growth or ossification centers in children, beginning with necrosis followed by regeneration or recalcification
B. Classification
   1. *Legg-Calvé-Perthes disease* (see foregoing)
   2. *Köhler's disease:* Osteochrondrosis of tarsal navicular bone

3. *Osgood-Schlatter disease:* Osteochondrosis of tibial tuberosity as consequence of partial avulsion of infrapatellar tendon from cartilaginous tibial tuberosity
4. *Syndig-Larsen disease:* Osteochondrosis of patella

C. Manifestations

Mild local tenderness, pain, swelling, motor disability

D. Diagnosis

X-ray examination

E. Treatment

Refer to orthopaedist

SCOLIOSIS (Figs. 112, 113)

A. Definition

Lateral curvature of spine

B. Causes
1. Idiopathic (most prevalent)
2. Congenital vertebral abnormalities
3. Neuromuscular diseases (*i.e.,* poliomyelitis, muscular dystrophy)
4. Spinal irradiation
5. Tuberculosis
6. Neurofibromatosis
7. Marfan's syndrome

C. Diagnosis

X-ray examination

D. Treatment
1. Mild involvement requires no treatment
2. Moderate involvement may be treated with back brace (Milwaukee brace)
3. Severe involvement requires surgical correction

E. Prognosis

Untreated, disorder may lead to spinal cord injury

DISLOCATION OF HEAD OF RADIUS

A. General Considerations
1. Referred to as "mad mother syndrome," "nursemaid's elbow"
2. Usually occurs as result of child being suddenly jerked by the hand
3. Peak age incidence 2–5 years

B. Manifestations
1. Immediate but not persistent pain in elbow
2. Inability to supinate forearm
3. Child usually holds entire arm close to body and refuses to move it

C. Diagnosis
1. History and manifestations
2. X-ray examination normal

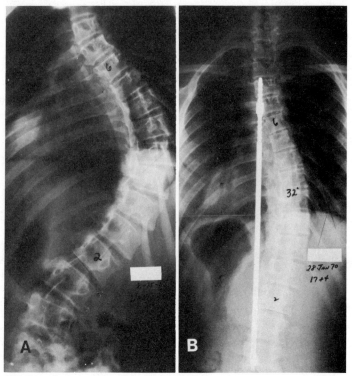

Fig. 112. Severe right thoracic, left lumbar "idiopathic" scoliosis **(A)** corrected with a Harrington rod and posterior spine fusion **(B)**. Surprisingly, these patients have minimal disability and can lead a full life complete with sports activities and no interference with pregnancy or delivery. (*Lovell WW, Winter RB (eds): Pediatric Orthopaedics, Vol. 2. Philadelphia, J. B. Lippincott, 1978*)

D. Treatment
  1. Reduction easily accomplished. With elbow in extension, head of radius is firmly pressed while forearm is supinated
  2. Reduction followed by prompt relief and child is immediately willing to move extremity in all directions
  3. Parents should be warned not to lift child by his/her hands since condition is prone to recur

MISCELLANEOUS DISORDERS

A. Pectus Excavatum (Funnel Chest): Indentation of lower part of sternum. Surgical correction for cosmetic reasons or if compression causes cardiopulmonary embarrassment

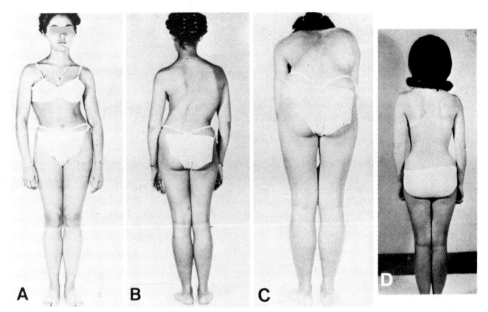

Fig. 113. Idiopathic scoliosis in a girl 15 years 3 months old. **(A)** Front view. Note tilting of the body toward the right and prominence of the left iliac crest. **(B)** Back view. Note right thoracic and left lumbar curvature and prominence of right scapula and high right shoulder. **(C)** Back view with spine flexed showing prominence of right upper back (razorback deformity). **(D)** Back view four years after an arthrodesis of part of the dorsal and lumbar spine, showing essentially normal alignment of the trunk. (*Shands AR et al: In Shirkey HC (ed): Pediatric Therapy, p 1152. Saint Louis, C. V. Mosby, 1975*)

B. Pectus Carinatum (Pigeon Breast): Protuberant sternum. No treatment indicated
C. Craniosynostosis: Premature closure of cranial sutures. If severe, may require surgical correction because of possible cerebral damage or for cosmetic reasons
D. Achondroplasia (Chondrodystrophy): Disorder of cartilage beginning *in utero* and leading to type of dwarfism in which long bones are most severely affected. Large head, saddle nose, lordosis* are associated features
E. Acute Discitis
   1. A disease process of intervertebral disc. Is also known as benign osteitis of spine
   2. Average age of onset, 3 years
   3. Etiology uncertain (trauma, viral, bacterial origins considered)
   4. Signs and symptoms include walking with spine rigid, difficulty in walking or standing, back pain, abdominal pain
   5. Diagnosis established by radionuclide bone scan (technetium or gallium) or by roentgenogram
   6. Needle aspiration of vertebral disc has revealed presence of staphylococci on culture in some cases

* See Glossary

7. Treatment consists of bed rest. Use of antibiotic therapy still controversial but probably indicated

BIBLIOGRAPHY

Chung S: Diseases of the developing hip. Pediatr Clin North Am 24:857–870, 1977

Hoekelman RA et al: Principals of Pediatrics. Health Care of the Young. New York, McGraw-Hill, 1978

Klein HA: Back deformities. Pediatr Clin North Am 24:857–870, 1977

McDale W: Bow legs and knock knees. Pediatr Clin North Am 24:825–841, 1977

Rudolph AM, Barnett HL, Einhorn AH: Pediatrics. New York, Appleton-Century-Crofts, 1977

Staheli LT: Torsional deformity. Pediatr Clin North Am 24:799–812, 1977

Vaughan VC III, McKay RJ, Nelson WE: Nelson Textbook of Pediatrics. Philadelphia, W. B. Saunders, 1975

23

Miscellaneous Disorders

CYSTIC FIBROSIS

A. Definition

An autosomal recessive disease characterized by dysfunction of exocrine (mainly mucous) glands

B. Incidence

1. In Caucasians, 1 in 1600 live births
2. All ethnic groups affected
3. in blacks, approximately 1 in 16,000
4. Rare in Orientals

C. Etiology and Pathogenesis

1. Cause unknown
2. Abnormally viscous secretions of mucus are basis for the various manifestations
3. Process may begin in fetus with consequent meconium ileus
4. The thick mucous secretions may inspissate pancreas, bile ducts, lungs (interfering with mucociliary transport)

D. Meconium Ileus

1. General Considerations

      a. Is earliest clinical manifestation of cystic fibrosis (5–10% of patients)

      b. Almost all cases are due to cystic fibrosis

  2. Definition

      Obstruction of small intestine (usually in area of ileocecal valve) with putty-like grayish meconium

  3. May result in perforation with meconium peritonitis

  4. Manifestations

      a. Abdominal distention

      b. Vomiting

      c. Failure to pass meconium

  5. Diagnosis

      a. Intestinal obstruction established by x-ray examination

      b. Positive family history for cystic fibrosis is helpful

  6. Treatment

      a. Gastrografin enemas may relieve uncomplicated case

      b. Surgery required in almost 50%

E. General Features

  1. General Considerations

      a. May appear to be perfectly normal or may appear to be chronically ill

      b. With severe involvement, have barrel chest, cough, dyspnea, cyanosis, clubbing of nails

      c. Abdominal distention, hypoproteinemia, edema, rectal prolapse may occur

      d. *Voracious appetite in a severely malnourished child with a troublesome cough* must suggest diagnosis of cystic fibrosis

  2. Gastrointestinal System

      a. Stools may be loose or may be large, foul, and fatty (due to fat intolerance because of pancreatic insufficiency)

      b. Glucose intolerance may occur in older patients

      c. Alterations in pancreas may result in chemical diabetes

      d. Cirrhosis and portal hypertension may occur in older patients

  3. Pulmonary System

      a. Lungs normal at birth

      b. Lungs are prone to infection, initially with *Staphylococcus aureus* and later with *Pseudomonas aeruginosa*

      c. Intercurrent viral infections not uncommon

      d. Pneumonia common but rarely due to pneumococcus

      e. Atelectasis, bronchitis, bronchiectasis, common

      f. Pneumothorax and pulmonary hemorrhage are ominous complications

  4. Genitourinary System

      a. 95% of males are infertile because of structural defects in vas deferens, epididymus, seminal vesicles

      b. Calcified prostatic secretions not uncommon

      c. Many females cannot become pregnant, possibly because of viscous cervical secretions or cervical plug

5. Cardiovascular System
   a. Bronchopulmonary shunts secondary to development of large bronchial collaterals
   b. Cor pulmonale (right ventricular hypertrophy secondary to severe pulmonary disease)
      1. May eventually cause heart failure and death
      2. Treatment aimed at pulmonary disorder and, if congestive heart failure is present, should include decongestive measures
F. Diagnosis
   1. Clinical manifestations
   2. Family history
   3. Roentgenogram of chest
   4. Sweat test establishes diagnosis
      a. Sodium and chloride almost always elevated
      b. Sweat chloride usually more than 60 mEq/liter
G. Treatment
   1. Pancreatic insufficiency
      a. Adequate caloric intake
      b. Pancreatic enzymes [pancrelipase (Viokase or Cotazyme)]
      c. Multivitamins including vitamin E
   2. Pulmonary disorder
      a. Chest physical therapy to loosen secretions
      b. Antibiotic therapy when infection is present
         1. Includes wide variety of agents: dicloxacillin, cephalexin monohydrate (Keflex), erythromycin, clindamycin hydrochloride (Cleocin), sulfisoxazole (Gantrisin) for staphylococcal infections
         2. Colistin, gentamycin, tobramycin, carbenicillin for *Pseudomonas aeruginosa*
         3. Choice of antibiotic and duration of treatment must be individualized and varies considerably in different cystic fibrosis centers
   3. Intermittent hospitalization frequently necessary
H. Prognosis
   1. Pulmonary process usually dominates and determines clinical course
   2. Mean survival now 12–20 years
   3. Survival beyond 30 years extremely rare

SUDDEN INFANT DEATH SYNDROME (SIDS)

A. Definition
   Sudden death in any infant in whom death was not expected and autopsy examination fails to reveal cause
B. General Considerations
   1. Generally in good health prior to death

2. Worldwide in distribution
3. Peak incidence 2–4 months of age
4. Rare after 1 year of age
5. More frequent in males
6. More common in blacks than in whites
7. Increased risk with low-birth-weight infants

C. Etiology
1. Cause unknown—probably multifactorial
2. Many hypotheses, none yet proved

MARFAN'S SYNDROME

Definition
A connective tissue disorder characterized by tall stature, arachnodactyly,* aortic dilation. An autosomal dominant disease

MUCOPOLYSACCHARIDOSES

A. Definition
A group of diseases characterized by excess tissue storage and urinary excretion of mucopolysaccharides

B. Types
1. *Hurler's syndrome (Type I):* Onset 6–18 months. Coarse facies, cloudy cornea, stiff joints, kyphosis,* valvular heart disease. Autosomal recessive disease
2. *Hunter's syndrome (Type II):* Onset 2–4 years. Course facies, stiff joints, kyphosis rare, deafness, X-linked recessive disease
3. *Sanfillippo's syndrome (Type III):* Mildly coarse facies, clear cornea, mildly stiff joints, no kyphosis, mentally deficient. Autosomal recessive disease
4. *Morquio's syndrome (Type IV):* Onset 1–3 years. Coarse facies, cloudy cornea, stiff joints, flattened vertebrae, *severe* kyphosis. Autosomal recessive disease
5. *Scheie's syndrome (Type V):* Broad mouth, cloudy cornea, stiff joints, no kyphosis. Autosomal recessive disease
6. *Maroteaux-Lamy syndrome (Type VI):* Onset 1–3 years. Coarse facies, cloudy cornea, stiff joints, kyphosis. Autosomal recessive disease

TREACHER-COLLINS SYNDROME
(MANDIBULOFACIAL DYSOSTOSIS)

An autosomal dominant disease characterized by malar and mandibular hypoplasia, defects of lower eyelid, antimongoloid slant to eyes, malformed external ears

* See Glossary

PIERRE ROBIN SYNDROME

A congenital abnormality characterized by micrognathia, glossoptosis,* cleft palate

PRADER-WILLI SYNDROME

A disease complex characterized by obesity, hypogenitalism, hypotonia, mental deficiency, short stature, diabetes mellitus

STURGE-WEBER SYNDROME

A disease complex characterized by port-wine hemangioma of face, hemangiomas of meninges, seizures, unilateral glaucoma. Mental deficiency usually present. May have intracranial calcifications

NEUROFIBROMATOSIS

An autosomal dominant disease characterized by bone lesions, neurofibromas, café au lait spots, tendency to develop intracranial tumors and pheochromocytoma

TUBEROUS SCLEROSIS

An autosomal dominant disease characterized by pink or brownish facial skin nodules (adenoma sebaceum), seizures, mental deficiency. May have intracranial calcifications

BIBLIOGRAPHY

Arnon SS et al: Infantile botulism—? One cause of sudden infant death syndrome. Lancet 1:1273–1276, 1978

Hoekelman RA et al: Principals of Pediatrics. Health Care of the Young. New York, McGraw-Hill, 1978

Kelly DH et al: The role of the QT interval in the sudden infant death syndrome. Circulation 55:633–635, 1977

Rudolph AM, Barnett HL, Einhorn AH: Pediatrics. New York, Appleton-Century-Crofts, 1977

Scott OJ et al: Respiratory viruses and sudden infant death syndrome (SIDS). Br Med J 2:12–13, 1978

Shwachman H: Cystic fibrosis. In Pediatrics Update. Reviews for Physicians, 1:215–231, 1979

Vaughan VC III, McKay RJ, Nelson WE: Nelson Textbook of Pediatrics. Philadelphia, W. B. Saunders, 1975

* See Glossary

Glossary

Acholic Stool.   Stool free of bile.

Acrocyanosis.   Cyanosis and coolness of hands and feet.

Alopecia Totalis.   Total baldness of areas normally containing hair.

Aniridia.   Absence of iris.

Arachnodactyly.   Condition in which fingers and toes are abnormally slender and long.

Arnold-Chiari Malformation.   Congenital anomaly in which cerebellum and medulla oblongata project through the foramen magnum. May be associated with many defects (*i.e.,* spina bifida, meningomyelocele).

Athetosis.   Ceaseless, involuntary, slow, writhing movements, more pronounced in hands.

Atrial Septostomy.   Procedure designed to enlarge foramen ovale and increase shunting. Consists of ripping atrial septum by passing balloon catheter through foramen ovale during cardiac catheterization and rapidly withdrawing it.

Beckwith's Syndrome.   Familial disease manifested by omphalocele, macroglossia, cytomegaly of fetal adrenal cortex, hyperplasia of kidney and pancreas, hypoglycemia, and gigantism.

Blepharospasm. Tonic contraction of orbicularis oculi muscle, causing partial or complete closure of eyelids.

Brachycephaly. Small head.

Brushfield Spots. White specks of iris seen in Down's syndrome.

Café Au Lait Spots. Pigmented areas of skin of variable sizes and shapes.

Carrying Angle. Angle formed between arm and forearm when forearm is extended (angle is prominent in Turner's Syndrome)

Catarrhal. Pertaining to inflammation of a mucous membrane with a free discharge.

Cerebral Vascular Accident. Sudden spells of hyperpnea, deep cyanosis, possible loss of consciousness.

Chordee. Ventral bend of penis.

Choreoathetosis. Disorder marked by involuntary, irregular, jerking and slow, writhing movements.

Chvostek Sign. Temporary spasm of facial muscles induced by tapping on branches of facial nerve (anterior to ear).

Claudication. Limping or lameness. Intermittent is common form manifested by onset of pain and weakness of leg upon walking that increases in severity upon further exercise. Patient asymptomatic at rest.

Colobomata. Congenital fissure or defect of eye (iris, sclera).

Coombs' Test. Detects presence of antibodies on red blood cells (direct) or in serum (indirect). Test is positive in Rh incompatibility.

Coryza. Acute inflammation of nasal mucous membranes with profuse nasal discharge.

Cover Test. Determines presence of phoria. Examiner has patient stare straight ahead and covers one eye. Deviation of other eye indicates phoria (each eye must be tested separately).

Cover-Uncover Test. Identical to cover test except after covering eye, examiner uncovers eye and watches for movement in that eye (only one eye need be tested).

Cubitus Valgus. Deviation of forearm away from midline.

Downey Cell. Atypical lymphocyte with larger than normal cytoplasmic to nuclear ratio and with cytoplasmic vacuoles.

Dysarthria. Difficulty in speaking (speech impediment).

Dysphagia. Difficulty in swallowing.

Eisenmenger Complex. Any congenital heart disease in which pulmonary vascular disease causes a left-to-right shunt to reverse.

Ejection Click. High-pitched clicking sound, occurring shortly after first heart sound. Thought to be due to sudden distention of dilated pulmonary artery or aorta.

Enanthem. Mucous membrane eruption.

Encephalocele. Congenital hernia of brain through opening of skull.

Enophthalmos. Retraction of eye into orbit (sunken eyeball).

Erythema Multiforme. Acute disorder of skin usually characterized by burning and pruritic macules and papules that may last for several days. May be accompanied by headache and gastrointestinal complaints.

Erythema Nodosum. Inflammatory disease of skin presenting with burning, pruritic, tender, bluish-red nodules. Lesions appear in successive patches lasting several weeks. Associated with sarcoidosis, histoplasmosis, coccidiomycosis, Yersinia infections, collagen vascular diseases, drug reactions.

Exophthalmos.   Abnormal protrusion of eyeball (bulging eye).

Fecalith.   Intestinal calculus composed of fecal matter.

Gallop.   Presence of extra heart sound (third or fourth). Upon auscultation, sounds are like those of a galloping horse.

Gavage.   Feeding through nasogastric tube in stomach.

Glabella.   Area between eyebrows.

Glossoptosis.   Structural condition in which tongue is retracted and displaced downward.

Guillain-Barré Syndrome.   Disorder characterized by bilateral ascending paralysis, usually following respiratory illness. Prolonged course with generally good prognosis.

Gumma.   Soft tumor seen in tertiary syphilis; composed of granulation tissue.

Gynecomastia.   Hypertrophy of male mammary glands.

Harrison's Groove.   Horizontal depression across lower chest corresponding to diaphragmatic attachment. Seen in children with chronic respiratory disease or rickets.

Hematemesis.   Blood in vomitus.

Heterochromia.   Presence of two colors in an area of the body (*e.g.*, iris) that should normally be of one color (*e.g.*, iris).

Holt-Oram Syndrome.   Autosomal dominant hereditary heart disease (atrial septal defect or ventricular septal defect) associated with skeletal abnormalities (hypoplastic thumb and short forearm).

Hutchinson Triad.   Diffuse keratitis, deafness (labyrinthine), and Hutchinson teeth (notched incisors, mulberry molars). Occurs in untreated congenital syphilis.

Hydrocele.   Circumscribed collection of fluid in tunica vaginalis of testis.

Hypertelorism.   Abnormal increase in the interorbital distance.

Hypoxic Episode.   Early morning episode in children with cyanotic heart disease characterized by hyperpnea, deepening cyanosis, and sometimes syncope and convulsions.

Incarceration.   Hernia that cannot be reduced. High probability of bowel strangulation and necrosis.

Ipsilateral.   Located on or pertaining to same side.

Janeway Lesions.   Small erythematous or hemorrhagic areas, usually located on palms or soles.

Kussmaul Respirations.   *Deep*, labored breathing.

Kyphosis.   Abnormal dorsal protrusion of vertebral column (humpback).

Laurence-Moon-Biedl Syndrome.   Characterized by hypogenitalism, retinitis pigmentosa, obesity, skull defects, mental retardation, and occasionally syndactyly.

Lesch-Nyhan Syndrome.   Rare X-linked condition characterized by mental retardation, self-mutilation of fingers and lips by biting, spastic cerebral palsy, impaired renal function, and hyperuricemia. Caused by deficiency of hypoxanthine-guanine phosphoribosyltransferase that causes defective purine metabolism.

Lordosis.   Ventral convexity of vertebral column.

Macrosomia. Large body size

Meconium. Dark green mucouslike substance present in intestine of mature fetus. Composed of amniotic fluid, intestinal secretions, and squamous cells.

Meconium Plug Syndrome. Lower colonic obstruction caused by small mass of hardened meconium. Evacuation of plug causes immediate relief.

Melena. Stools stained with blood pigments.

Micrognathia. Abnormally small jaw (receding chin).

Microphthalmia. Abnormally small eyes.

Miosis. Contraction of pupil.

Mongolian Spots. Bluish areas on back and sometimes extremities in dark-skinned babies (of no pathologic significance).

Myringitis. Inflammation of tympanic membrane.

Myringotomy. Surgical incision of posterior inferior portion of tympanic membrane. Releases fluid from middle ear and prevents spontaneous perforation.

Myxedema. Associated with hypothyroidism and consists of dry, nonpitting, waxy swelling of body with mucinous deposits in soft tissues.

Neonatal Tetany. A temporary dysfunction of calcium homeostasis due to or aggravated by the high phosphorus content of cow's milk.

Obtundation. State of lowered consciousness. Still responds to simple stimuli.

Oculogyric Crisis. Seen in epidemic encephalitis where eyeballs are fixed in one position (may last for minutes to hours).

Oligohydramnios. Less than 300 ml of amniotic fluid at term.

Oliguria. Decreased production of urine (less than 0.5 ml/kg/hr).

Opsiclonus. Nonrhythmic horizontal and vertical oscillations of eyes.

Orthoptics. Eye exercises designed to correct visual axes in patients with improperly coordinated binocular vision.

Osler Nodes. Small, raised, tender areas (usually bluish) occurring in pads of fingers or toes. Practically pathognomonic of subacute bacterial endocarditis.

Paraumbilical. Next to umbilicus but does not involve it.

Paresthesia. Burning or prickling sensation that may occur spontaneously or with light touch.

Pericardiocentesis. Puncture of pericardium in order to aspirate fluid from pericardial cavity.

Pica. Ingestion of unnatural foods (*e.g.*, stool, dirt, hair).

Polydipsia. Excessive thirst.

Polyhydramnios. Excess amniotic fluid.

Polyphagia. Excessive eating or voracious appetite.

Prader-Willi Syndrome. Obesity, mental retardation, hypogonadism, and hypotonia.

Proptosis. A bulging or forward displacement (usually refers to eye).

Ptosis. Drooping of upper eyelid, usually secondary to paralysis of third or sympathetic nerves.

Pulsus Alternans (Alternating Pulse). Peripheral pulses follow alternating weak–strong pattern without variation of ventricular cycle time.

Pulsus Paradoxus. Drop in systolic blood pressure greater than 20 mm Hg during inspiration (sign of cardiac tamponade).

Pyoderma Gangrenosum.   Circumscribed cutaneous ulcers with liquefying border associated with ulcerative colitis, regional enteritis, or rheumatoid arthritis.

Raynaud's Phenomenon.   Intermittent episodes of pallor of fingers and toes brought on by cold.

Retrolental Fibroplasia.   A retinopathy primarily in premature infants, usually precipitated by excess oxygen.

Rhagades.   Cracks, fissures, or small linear scars of skin. Usually occur around area subjected to frequent movement (*e.g.*, mouth).

Sandifer's Syndrome.   Hiatal hernia coexisting with twisting of neck and abnormal head position (torticollis). Torticollis presumably results from patient attempting to relieve pain secondary to gastroesophageal reflux.

Saucerization.   Excavation of tissue to form shallow depression to facilitate drainage of infected areas of bone.

Schilling Test.   A test for absorption of vitamin B_{12}. Normally, radioactive vitamin B_{12}, administered orally, is absorbed but not excreted in the urine, since it is bound by the tissues and the blood proteins. When followed by parenterally administered nonradioactive vitamin B_{12}, the previously absorbed radioactive vitamin is "flushed out" and can be detected in the urine in significant quantities. In pernicious anemia, since the orally administered vitamin B_{12} is poorly absrobed, none can be "flushed out" of the tissues, and only a trace (not more than 2%) will appear in the urine with the provocative parenteral administration of the vitamin.

Scotch Tape Test.   Sticky surface of scotch tape is applied to anus before bath in morning. Tape is then placed sticky side down on glass slide and preparation is examined microscopically for ova.

Septostomy.   Incision of a septum. Customarily used in relation to the atrial septum of the heart where the septum is ripped by a balloon catheter to provide cross-circulation in complete transposition of the great arteries. This procedure is called the Rashkind procedure.

Setting-Sun Sign.   Downward displacement of iris so that it appears to "set" beneath lower lid. Sclera is visible between upper lid and iris.

Sideroblastic Anemia.   Nucleated red cells with hemosiderin granules surrounding the nucleus. Basic defect may be abnormality of iron or heme metabolism.

Somnambulism.   Sleep walking.

Strangulation.   Cessation of circulation due to compression.

Sturge-Weber Syndrome.   Congenital disorder characterized by nevus flammeus of face, angiomas of leptomeninges and choroid, and late glaucoma. Frequently associated with intracranial calcifications, mental retardation, contralateral hemiplegia, and epilepsy.

Syndactyly.   Persistent webbing between adjacent fingers or toes such that they are partially or completely attached.

Systolic Click.   A high-pitched ejection sound that occurs shortly after the first heart sound. It is attributed to forceful opening of thickened semilunar valves or to sudden distention of an enlarged pulmonary artery or aorta.

Tarsus of Eyelid.   Connective tissue plate forming framework of eyelid.

Telangiectasis.   Red area caused by dilated blood vessels. Area blanches on palpation.

Testicular Feminization Syndrome. Extreme form of male pseudohermaphroditism with female external genitalia and secondary sexual development but with presence of testes and absence of uterus and tubes.

Thrill. Palpable vibration over precordium associated with *loud* systolic or diastolic murmurs (grades IV–VI).

Tinnitus. Ringing or buzzing noise in ear.

Trendelenberg Position. Supine position with head tilted downward.

Trousseau's Sign. Clinical test for tetany, based on production of carpal spasm elicited by constriction of upper arm. When positive, carpal spasm occurs.

Tuttle Test. Acid is introduced into stomach and acidity is then measured in lower esophagus. Presence of acid in lower esophagus is positive test and indicates gastroesophageal reflux.

Vernix Caseosa. A cheesy appearing substance, composed of desquamated epithelial cells and sebum, that covers the skin of the fetus.

Vitiligo. Depigmented areas of skin of variable shape and size.

Volvulus. Obstruction of bowel secondary to twisting of intestinal segment on mesenteric attachment. High association of vascular compromise and secondary infarction.

Index

Numerals followed by an *f* indicate a figure; *t* following a page number indicates tabular material.